From a Branch:
ALZHEIMER

# From a Branch: ALZHEIMER

## Celia Álvarez Fresno

Translation from the original Spanish
by Nicholas Kleinerman

Alexandria Library
MIAMI

ISBN: 978-1477645406

http://celiaalvarezfresno.blogspot.com/

This book also is also available for purchase on Amazon Kindle

www.alexlib.com

# Contents

For you, caring for a patient with Alzheimer's.

And above all, for you... for that gaze of yours, where you hide your memories, those memories that were taken from you by such a terrible disease.

# The author's perceptions

Once the disease is detected, we must be prepared, for the periods of adaptation to the new situation are hard.

At first, there is disbelief, and you ask yourself: "Why him?" or "Why her?"

Really, this is an easy question to answer: "Because we are all alive and anything can happen to us."

Therefore, rather than deny the obvious, you must face the situation and carry on, full of hope. You must keep your feet on the ground – do not live with the false hope that everything will be the same, that he or she will recover their faculties.

From my own experience, I can tell you that if you go along preparing yourself mentally, it is not so terrible. When things progress little by little, we have the time to focus positively enough on what will be.

I focused on the day to day. I did not think about every day, about every situation, nor did I think about what would become of her or of us. No. If you wish to climb a mountain, you must concentrate your efforts on a single footstep, and you must concentrate on knowing where you are placing your foot. In this way, it is quite possible for you to reach the peak. If you only concentrate on the goal, it is likely that you will never get there.

The same happens with Alzheimer's.

You must be strong and must understand that this is the disease of goodbyes and of multiple deaths. And it is this way because with each step they leave something behind.

One day they will lose their present history; but you must go on remembering how they were. Emphasize the pleasant moments they have lived; and, above all, praise all the positive things they accomplished during that period of their lives now forgotten. Speak to them; recall the names of family and friends, and the names of all those who have meant something special to him or her. Simply mentioning the name of a dog or animal they may have had will make them smile.

They have lost their memories but you are still there to narrate their story.

One day they will no longer recognize you. Don't let that bother you, even though a moment like this is indescribably difficult, because, inside, they still know who you are. One thing is the mind, and another, very different, thing is the heart.

One day they will become moody, even violent and they will try to exert their will. Then, use all the arguments available; at this moment their minds still retain a certain degree of lucidity, because the disease is still at an early stage. Try to convince them of what is correct and what is not. If you manage to restore calm, cheer them up, give them a kiss and hug them. If you cannot restore calm, try to explain to them that the situation is more than you can handle. Many times you will be surprised at the affection that comes out from hiding behind their apparent incoherence.

One day they will no longer be able to feed themselves; don't fret, because you will feed them and give them their favorite food. Though they may not be able to hold utensils, they do know how to enjoy what you give them.

Laugh with them when they are being funny. At first, and even after the disease has progressed, they say things that are funny and out of place. Don't feel funny about laughing along with them, and let them know that you find this new facet of theirs charming. Let them know that before they were more serious. They enjoy it very much when the people around them are happy.

One day they will no longer be able to walk, and you will let them know how lucky they are, that now they get around on wheels, in the very chair in which they are sitting. And that this is a good thing for everyone, because it is safer, and that they have already walked enough.

They will be afraid of water; you, little by little, with a damp sponge, will let them once again feel the pleasant sensations of water upon their body.

It is a disease full of fears and insecurities. A simple shoe will perhaps seem threatening to them, or they may run, terrified, from a simple comb.

Insecurity, loneliness and uncertainty are always present in them.

Never forget to look them in the eyes. Many times their gaze is vacant. And it is not that they are not there; simply, there are two worlds available to them. They remove themselves from one world to enter into the other, into a world which is new for them. But it will surprise you how many times their gaze is the same as always.

Never yell at them, because their gaze will turn violent. They show a terrible fear of everything. They feel so alone that it is necessary to hug them, to give them kisses, to pamper them and comfort them with tender words and love.

Put your face next to theirs, and most probably they will give you a loud kiss. Keep in mind that feelings never die.

For that reason, I am certain that, despite their apparent absence, there exists a world of perceptions, of sensations, and of life from which we should learn.

The journey is a difficult one, but it can be made sweeter by accepting the reality of the situation, and by helping them, with your love, to scale the difficult summit which circumstances have forced them to take on.

# I

A beautiful book is a victory won on all the
battlefields of human thought

Honoré de Balzac

Laura is suffering from Alzheimer's. She is still young, only fifty-six. Too young to let the history of her life slip away. Too young to let go of life itself.

At the onset of her disease, some time ago, the lapses in memory began to occur daily. And her situation took a turn for the worse when she found herself, at times, unable to remember what certain objects were used for, familiar objects which she had held in her hands so many times.

"Mom. You told me today we would go out when I got home from work... and you haven't even gotten ready. You look a mess. Why? Is anything wrong?"

"No, sweetheart. What could be wrong? I simply didn't remember. Enough, already. Let me get ready, and then we'll go."

When Ana, her daughter, began to notice some odd behavior, she became frightened... maybe that doctor, a while back, had been on to something with his diagnosis.

And from that moment on, she became aware of her mother's inexplicable and unpredictable reactions.

"Why are you spinning the silverware like that?"

"What do you mean? I'm spinning the silverware? Your head must be spinning. Sweetheart, really... What is this? What do I do with this?"

Or, right after finishing a meal, she would assert that she hadn't had a bite to eat. At nighttime, she would think it was daytime. And when it was day, she thought it was night.

"I just got a little disoriented, sweetheart."

Ana will forever remember that sad day when she arrived home and her mother was nowhere to be found.

"Hello? Oh, yes, excuse me. It's just that I am very frightened. It's my mother... my mother is not at home. I came home and she wasn't here. In the afternoon, at this hour, it's strange to come home and not find her here... I'm afraid for the worst. That's why I thought of calling 911, that's you, correct?"

"Yes... I know, maybe she got to talking with someone and lost track of the time. But she doesn't have a cell phone with her, and I think... I think... it looks like she is in the early stages of Alzheimer's. She becomes disoriented easily. Today... today, I'm afraid for the worst."

"Yes. She may be wearing a dress with a floral print; the truth is I don't know. She's thin, blonde... rather tall. No, she doesn't wear glasses. I just noticed that... she even left her keys here..."

"Yes... she likes the park a lot. Yes, near the beach. Please... I'll go out right now too."

"Yes... yes... let's keep in contact, please. I am scared to death. If anything happens to her... I will never forgive myself."

"Okay, I'll try to calm down. Yes..."

In the end, she turned up, sitting on a bench by the rose garden. She looked quite happy, and when she saw her daughter arrive, she didn't even blink an eye. She simply said:

"Sit down here next to me. I was waiting for you."

Sometimes, in the middle of the night, she would find her in her room, ready to go outside. Sometimes dressed impeccably and other times with three or four jackets on.

"Mom, it's time to get into bed. You can't get up now... Don't you see it is nighttime? Look out the window, see for yourself."

"Have some respect for your elders, and move aside. Let me by, because you are becoming rude and unbearable. I am going to have to take some serious measures with you."

Yes. And even though things started out this way, she did still have completely normal days. Days when it did not seem possible that she could be in the middle of a degenerative process. But other days...

"For God's sake, someone please do something about these animals that have gotten into the living room."

"They're on TV. They are not going to get in the living room."

"They're on TV? You really must have lost it. Don't you see that they are getting in everywhere?"

Other times, she would have a book in her hands. She would read it, but she could not follow it. No, it's not that she wouldn't make the effort, and in fact she often seemed to be trying, but she just was not capable of concentrating her attention on anything.

"Mom... What are you reading?"

"It's... a... a book. Can't you see that?"

"And have you read much of it?"

"Yes... I think so."

"What's it about?"

"It's about.... about..."

During this phase, Laura was subject to frequent mood swings. Now yes... now no... one moment, she would love freely, openly, and she would cover you with kisses and caresses; then, suddenly, she would cast sidelong glances at that person who just a few minutes before was the object of her unreserved affection and trust, this person having now become, in her mind, a possible traitor, a thief scheming to get at that purse she was now clutching at her side.

She did not show an interest in anything. Or perhaps, yes, for a brief moment, only to then tumble into a feeling of boredom which grew heavier over time. Her distant memories, of years ago, still lived on in her mind. The same could not be said for her ability to recall more recent memories; she could not remember what she had had for breakfast today or with whom she had spoken while crossing the street.

She would soon pass through a number of different phases, each one distinct, though not necessarily more bitter. And, perhaps, at the end of the path that lay ahead, a path so difficult to climb, the precipice leveled off into flatlands...

Laura was an attractive woman, with green eyes and golden hair. She would often touch her hand to her head in an unmistakable sign of coquettishness, and she would stroke that hair of which she was so proud. Her eyes were full of sweetness. Now, since she had started coming to terms with her disease, they began to grow dim. Or, perhaps it would be more correct to say that her gaze had retreated to places hidden deep within her, to return later on. She was slim, and she had maintained that special elegance that had been bestowed upon her. All her life, she had walked quickly; she had seemed to always be in such a hurry to get everywhere, though this was not the case. She held her head high and her attitude perhaps seemed arrogant, but in reality she was not so.

Today Laura asked repeatedly where the living room was; she said it was not the same one as always, that someone had changed the decor and that that vase was pitiful. That yesterday it had smelled of blue and today... and today, it didn't even have a smell.

Her daughter had considered sending her to a day center, because she was afraid of what might happen to her when she was by herself, even though she was still in the early stages, as confirmed by the doctors looking after her. Helena, the woman who had, for some time, been cleaning and taking care of the house, was only there for a few hours. And so, Ana was trying to find a place that would take her mother while she was at work.

"Yes. Here, we have sufficient staff to take care of your mother. Of course, you can come visit our facilities... Our hours are from nine to five in the afternoon. A shuttle bus will come by your home each day to pick her up, and our staff will take care of her all day, including on the way here and home again."

"What activities do you offer? What I mean is... are they all together doing the same activities, or does it depend on the degree of their illness...?"

"Of course each one is in the place which best suits him or her. Your mother, from what you have told me, is still well... though not well enough to be carry out her day-to-day on her own. In cases such as hers, they do different activities; handicrafts... reading... painting... and they are with others who are at the same stage as she is. It's the best thing, because, otherwise, contact with others who are already suffering with the disease would make them feel out of place ..."

"Okay, I will call you back later – I have to see how I am going to be able to do this. I'm an only child, and really her only family... it's really hard. My mother has a lot of friends, but I don't want to burden anybody with a problem that, obviously... is my problem."

"I understand. Whatever decision you make, she is always welcome. From what you have told me, she may still experience a reasonable level of normality for some time yet. It's not strange to find that somewhat "different" attitude present in almost everyone at some moment in their lives. And those tend to be transitory situations. Give it some careful thought. We will be here to help. Rest assured."

"Thank you."

But Laura has a story, and her story will never be erased, because it is written in the memory of the Absolute; in the Archives of some hidden place of thought. In the prized box of her memories, which she carries on her lap.

# II

**Over time, time changes.**

Pierre Ronsard

She liked to see herself there in the distance, in her childhood, when she would chase about the meadows, taking in new sensations, with glittering lights all about her. She liked to linger there, among those marvelous memories which smelled of her parents; and then she would hug that treasure as tightly as she could, until she reached that first time, that first moment when she became aware of herself.

Curiously, her senses were responsible for steering her memory, and she could almost feel the wind on her face, coming from the fields, and the smell of hay, and the tinkling sound of the bells tied around the necks of the cows.

Even today, the smell of her father, Félix, brought the smell of green to her mind. "The smell of green?" Could colors, by themselves, really have a smell?

"You smell green, Dad."

"Sweetheart, listen... I smell like the field, and since it is green, you think the color green has its own smell. But it isn't like that, baby. I smell of Nature because we live in her, do you see?"

Even today, even though they told her when she was five years old that colors did not have any smell, she was convinced otherwise.

After all, didn't that man, the one with the dark raincoat who would sometimes pass by without lifting his head while he going up the meadow, didn't he smell black? And that woman who was forever with her cigarette, with the bits of paper and tobacco which stuck to her lips and never fell off even when she opened her mouth to talk on and on, didn't she smell gray?

Yes.

Whatever they might say, colors had a smell. She had always known it. And when she insisted on proving that it was true, her parents would offer to make a deal with her: "Sweetheart, if you want to, believe it to be so; but keep it to yourself, otherwise they are going to think you are out of your mind."

The farmhouse back then was surrounded by mountains and by dense groves; a small river flowed past. At the entrance to the house gleamed a 27, the numbers stenciled in blue. Perhaps that is why Laura insisted that the color blue smells of family, of the family home.

The house had two floors. On the upper floor, there were three bedrooms and a bathroom with a pitcher and a ceramic washbasin with different colored flowers painted on it. To access this floor you would go up a flight of stairs made of chestnut. Along the middle of the stairs, years and years of footsteps had left a slight groove. And there was the dining room, where Laura, one day, when she was five, admired her mother's beauty; she could still remember the moment perfectly:

Her mother, Ana, was up on a chair, struggling to hang a lace curtain up over the window, while Laura was on the floor, playing with a simple, shapeless doll with stiff arms and legs; she was, in fact, at that moment imitating the way the doll stretched out her hands and feet. However, as she was an impatient girl, that game usually did not last too long. She loved to dress up her doll with the dresses her mother would sew for her. But, what she liked most were the rag dolls and little horses that would sometimes appear suddenly, when she had lost a tooth or had been a good girl. And always, when that gift arrived, her heart would give a leap, and she would hug and kiss those unexpected toys.

While she was absorbed in playing with her doll, sitting on the floor and imitating her rigid posture, she heard a loud bang and saw the chair lying on its side on the floor, and her mother was saying to her:

"Laura, don't be frightened, it's nothing... I'm fine. What a fall!"

The girl moved like a shot to her mother's side and began caressing her face. Then she asked:

"Mom, are you an angel?"

"The things you say, baby... me, an angel... for God's sake, don't blaspheme."

"You're the most beautiful of anyone I know. What is 'blaspheme'?"

"Something you must avoid doing as long as you live, little lady."

"And what is 'avoid'?"

"Listen... as you go along in life, you'll learn these things, little by little. Don't be in such a hurry."

She always remembered those moments, just like she remembered her mother's soft and melodious voice announcing every morning that breakfast was on the table... her mother, who smelled of laundry blue.

And she smelled of laundry blue because, one day, she discovered some blue-colored balls in a small white bag.

"What's this?"

"Laundry blue."

"And what's it for?"

"When the clothes have been washed, these diluted balls are placed in the water with them, and the white colors turn a little blue. It's the remedy for all white garments."

"What does diluted mean? It's a really funny word."

23

"It means dissolved."

"And what does...?"

"Baby, for God's sake, be quiet, you're driving me crazy all day with all your questions..."

"Why don't I have the same name as you? Lots of girls in my class, they have the same name as their moms, but not me."

"Sweetheart, you have a beautiful name."

"Well, I like Ana better. Like you."

"What can we do? It can't be helped."

All during her life she had often thought about how she would have liked to have had brothers and sisters:

As time went by, and in response to Laura's questions about herself and about the possible brothers and sisters she never had, her mother told her that when she was born, there were serious complications, and that she almost lost her life giving birth to her. This was not at all unusual, considering the time period and, above all, out in the country, where women would give birth at home, assisted by a midwife, who was really no more than the woman on call who had certain skills in that area.

She remembered the smell of butter and toast, which still lingered in her senses and so well defined; even now, after so many years, it was as if those breakfasts around the wooden table, and everything around it, were today.

Every day unfolded the same way. Everything followed the same routine. Very early in the morning, Alfredo would arrive and set about milking the cows and helping Laura's father.

Alfredo was a big man, and very serious. He never said a word, and one time, when Laura was asking him about this and that, he answered, in a monotonous tone:

"Leave me alone. I have too much work to do, kid. Go ask your parents, they were able to go to school."

He would work all morning, and later, when he arrived with the wagon full of grass, that moment – and no other – was the moment which marked the time to leave for school. It was as though he wore a hidden watch, so that he wouldn't get distracted for even a minute.

"Mommy, Alfredo is coming and I'm not ready yet."

"No, baby, today is Sunday, and on Sunday we do other things. On Sunday we have to go to mass."

"I don't want to go, Mommy. Can't you see it's dark in there? Besides, it's boring."

"But, how many times have you told me you love the smell of the church?"

And then, from among the memories of yesteryear, Laura could smell the church; she smelled the incense that she used to like so much, that smell of white. Yes, churches smell white, even when they are dark and windowless.

It all seemed as if it weren't yesterday; the sounds were so intense in her ears, the stone wheel of the Mill, alongside the house, grinding up corn, she could hear it right now. Laura observed how that immense stone ground the cereal; then she roared with laughter while she stirred her coffee in the small hours of the morning.

Yes, she laughed because she was remembering her childhood escapades; Laura used to love to slip away from the others and climb the small dam with its cascading slopes in order, finally, to use her own force to turn the great round stone wheel.

"If you climb up there again, by yourself, without permission, you'll be punished and have to stay in all Sunday."

"I won't do it again, I promise."

But that wasn't so, and her fondness for doing what was 'not right' pursued her year after year. She was not fond of set ways, and she fought against everything she didn't like, with the goal of getting her own way.

That her house was just by the main road made her day more entertaining; though, if truth be told, Laura's imagination was filled to overflowing, and it didn't take much for her to put together a story which she would insist was true.

A horse used to pass by there – a Percheron – with broad legs and a wild mane, along with a lady who sold sweets and cotton candy, travelling from festival to festival. These country fairs, back then, were the only possible form of entertainment.

Laura would be in ecstasy over the treasures the woman would bring. She would run after the woman, this thick woman, whose hair was put up in a round bun on top of her head, the bun as round as the woman, and she would pull her father along by the hand, since she considered it would be easier to convince him to buy her all the things she liked so much.

"Daddy, I like everything the lady has brought."

"I know, sweetheart, but I can't buy everything. One thing, one little thing and no more. Sunday will come around again soon, you'll see, and I will treat you to another cotton candy."

And then she would be quite still, sitting under the Ash tree, savoring that sweet, sticky thing made of pink sugar which she held close to her round, little girl face while she stretched her tongue as far as she could to lick that tasty delicacy. The color pink had the smell of festivals. Of course it did.

Under that tree, she got over her tantrums, and when she wanted to hide it was her refuge. She liked its branches that shone in the sun and folded under the rain. She loved to watch when the wind made the crown roll and sway, and she would dream of one day being able to reach the top and sit amongst its branches.

The Ash tree was alongside the river, quite close to her house; close enough for her to make a shelter beside the tree, and she would even speak with it as if it were a friend. Even today, with these memories, the smell and taste of that sticky cotton candy reached her, and she smiled again and again, as the taste mixed with the smell of the fields and the pleasant memory of the leaves of the tree.

On stormy days, a swirl of lightning and black clouds could be seen over the clearing with the house with blue numbers.

Laura loved to watch the sky and see the flashes and the shapes and reflections. She enjoyed that interruption from the daily routine; because nothing as magical as that spectacle ever happened. And for such a restless young girl, for nothing to be happening was unacceptable.

She turned eight years old, and something occurred, something which did not leave her unaffected.

"Dad, I smell sadness."

"Oh, really? And... how does sadness smell, sweetheart, how does it smell? Come on, tell me."

"It smells empty here," she said, pointing to the pit of her stomach. "And it's brown. Sadness is brown."

"And why do you feel sad?"

"Because we have to leave this house, and I like it so much. And we live close to the school, and I like to walk up this way. I like it because Francisco and Teté come by for me, and from the other place I'll have to go by myself. I don't want to leave this place."

"Honey, it will be much nicer than this house. You'll be happy, you'll see."

And, today, Laura was convinced that she could smell sadness, because she felt something heavy, there, in the same place she could now see in her memories.

Her life changed when they moved to that other place; it was close to the first place, but with a house which to her seemed majestic. A house her father had ordered built; beautiful, spacious, grand, and full of light, with immense windows from which one could make out the neighboring country houses. Her bathroom seemed enormous, white... immaculately white. And the bedrooms, with the furniture from the previous house, were much nicer.

Here, the picture frames seemed to have a special shine. She could now see how the fat lady, the one seated, had her eyes half-shut, something she had never seen until then.

The house was located high up, quite close to the old house, halfway up the hillside and its steep fields. And of course – for how could it be otherwise – it was surrounded by green groves. The barn was a fair stretch from their home, and between the two structures there was a shed in which all the farming equipment was kept.

In the valley, the same small brook to which she had so often come, ran back for a few kilometers; in that brook she had many times observed leeches, toads, water striders – a kind of mosquito which always moved backwards without moving from its spot – and trout... such a sweet sound that brook made, songs of summer, washing up against the rocks. And later, when its waters grew murky and began to crest... then it said nothing anymore, because it was concentrating on flooding the valley and uprooting the crops.

"Oh! The peppers... the potatoes... all that work washed away downstream," her father would lament...

This happened again and again, one year after another, when the rains were most intense.

"Dad, why don't you plant farther up, where the water doesn't reach?"

And between laughs, she heard her father telling her: "Right there, that rich lowland area, by the river, that is where you can grow crops, because it is more fertile."

That word, 'fertile' stuck with Laura. It's interesting, she thought.

Even today, though many years had passed, Laura could still remember the smell of the river. It was a fresh smell, heavy with the smells of wet rock, of scrubbed soap, of eucalyptus leaves floating along on the water. She remembered her father so keenly, that green gaze, friendly gestures and beautiful hands that had so often, in another time, stroked her curly locks, ...

She could savor, off in the distance, the sweet taste of peaches and of embarrassed apples, which she imagined the ones that turned red to be ... they smelled so good... There were chickens pecking about here and there, cows mooing in their pastures, and Star, Navarra, or Mask returning to their stables, at night, to be milked. And Troski, the white and black dog, would howl when a neighbor passed away or bark when an intruder approached.

The house was not by the road, and for this reason the days were much more boring. Until... she turned ten. Ten. Her fetish period, because, on the day she turned ten, they gave her the most wonderful gift: a horse.

It was small, and it certainly did not have the most delicate hooves, nor did it carry itself elegantly; she learned how to ride. She used the animal's head to climb down again and again, and she hit the ground one day after the next. Yes. She fell many times, with no major consequences, since bones at that age are still supple, and the animal was not very tall. Little by little, she won him over and he won her over, and between them a bond formed which ended when the school year began and was reborn when summer started.

Laura could remember how it was when they first entered that flat in the city as well as how her first day at School was. The buildings in the city, the ones she recognized, had always seemed so immense to her, larger than she had ever imagined. The sky was not blue, and the clouds did not look like the ones she knew either. Everything was narrow, and the sky had a ruddy look to it, different; it wasn't like the other sky, wide, limitless. Here she could not entertain herself gazing at the shapes the clouds made for her. She could not run with her arms outstretched, looking like her little rubber doll, with the wind in her face.

Laura would cry a lot, and she would hear:

"That's enough already. You're going to get a good spanking if you don't stop howling like an animal. We will only be here during the school year. During vacation, we'll go back to the countryside; and you'll see, I can assure you, the day will come when you won't want to go. How I know it! You should keep in mind that in this life things are as they are, and many times we can't do what we want. Okay? Get it into your head, here things are different. Don't ever forget it."

"No. I won't forget it. Things are as they are."

And she went to her new bedroom, which she never grew to like, and she cried for a while. That flat in Gijón was so small, and it was nothing like that great big house so full of light. She didn't even like the kitchen, or her parent's room, or the living room and dining room. She felt like she was suffocating, and she wanted to get out through the window. A window which wasn't even a window, but, instead, was a balcony which didn't even have a single flower. Not a single flower!

# III

Today, Laura watched that past and became convinced that it was right now, even though so many years had passed. Yesterday and today mixed inevitably, and, in her thinking, memories and sensations diverged. The lamp, hanging there and shouting, was threatening her. She became afraid of the madness which seemed to have invaded her, and, at the same time, she felt sheltered and protected in that yesterday which had become today, and her today ... Where the hell was she? Who was she? She started to shake, to shake so hard that she forgot she was shaking, because the tangle had become so intense... She began to sweat. No sooner had the cold sweat completely invaded her, than she was suddenly herself again, expressing herself as if nothing had happened. The unfamiliar thoughts mixed together with the feelings of love and hate and emptiness, an emptiness which sent a shiver through her insides. Then, she yelled out, "Where are you? Mom, where are you?"

Suddenly, she was herself again; she remembered that her mother had gone away many years ago and was no longer alive. What is happening to me? What makes me think my mother could be here, if I know my parents died so many years ago?

"Ana! ... Where are you, baby?"

A now, a then, and an expression which raced across her soul, dragging her along... She sat down on the sofa. She began to perceive who she was really and where she was.

"Ma'am? What is wrong? Are you not feeling well? I was on the other side of the house, and I thought I heard you yelling ..."

"I was talking? You say I was yelling? No, of course I wasn't. Listen, Helena, I think you often talk nonsense. I don't want to say anything to my daughter, because she will certainly throw you out on the street, and I am a good person. I won't say anything to her; but, please, don't make up stories."

"Alright... maybe I was wrong; don't worry, it won't happen again."

One moment Laura was speaking quite coherently; and then, she was hurtling towards dark places in which there were death sentences, and people clamoring, and struggles between what was known and what was lost in that darkened part of her brain, which was reflected in her thoughts as if it were a broken mirror.

When her daughter got home, and Helena told her about what happened, the two women melted into each other's arms, aware of the hard road they had to travel.

# IV

Her mother thought that the girl had to look distinguished, and, since she liked flowers so much, she decided to buy her something at the 'Ten Prices', a variety shop which sold small flowers of every color.

"What is that for?"

"For the diadems. Each day I'll put a different colored flower in your hair, tucked under the diadem. Wait till you see how beautiful you'll look."

Quite annoyed, every morning she left the house wearing her gray uniform and that colorful diadem that really infuriated her.

The first day, she resigned herself to wearing the big crimson flower; but when she saw the shocked looks on the faces of her classmates she decided to hide the diadem in her schoolbag as soon as she left the house. The arguments that she was a princess and should be different were of little use to her after seeing how her classmates had looked at her in shock.

Little by little, she had to adapt to her new life, some kilometers away from the country. She missed the country life so much... The new center didn't look anything like the village school, where the schoolmistress, big, majestic, with her hair done up in a bun, knotted tightly against her neck, would recite a *good morning* to open that magic moment of morning encounters, in anticipation that the chorus of boys and girls would respond with a singsong, loud *Good mor-ning, Miss*, carefully enunciating each syllable while shouting it out.

That was the start of the school day. The chalkboard in the background, and the schoolmistress, with her rod in hand, in charge:

"I don't want to hear any one voice louder than the rest."

There were girls and boys of all ages, all together. Some used the blackboard and chalk, doodling and scribbling up and down and feeling like the masters of that piece of black slate; those were the smallest of the children, who were discovering their abilities for the first time. The older ones, the ones who were around ten years of age, would write their names and repeat the multiplication tables and the rules for spelling. There were cuffed ears and scoldings, but she put on a friendly face when a father or mother arrived with a basket full of vegetables from the garden, a token of appreciation for that woman they so highly valued and idolized; when it came to culture, all the mothers wished to be like her.

Right then and there, the teacher would turn sweet and would even smother the visiting parents' children with kisses. The children passing by her at that moment would behave as though they had just won some small prize to take back with them to their seats, and she would even smile at the rest, allowing the rod, her work companion, to rest behind that pulpit of sorts from where she would impart her knowledge. And then, the entire class would take advantage of the opportunity to do whatever they wanted, a whirlwind of activity set into motion by the temporary amnesty won by the visit.

There were no set hours. There were no specific days on which a certain evaluation of the pupil would be made; the pupil, when kissed by the lady with her hair tied up tightly to her neck in a bun, felt important, felt worthy in the eyes of his or her classmates, who drooled over the scene.

One day, Laura told the Mistress that her parents knew everything that she knew, and she was made to stand in the corner, with her arms held out, away from her sides, with a ton of books in each hand. "For being a smart aleck," she was told.

That schoolteacher was hard, but in those times, everything was hard, and the cuffed ears, the caning, it all seemed to be somewhat tolerable and, above all... healthy, necessary to live a good life. "Because the road of life is hard, and it is necessary to be strong," they would say.

# V

Past and present, a tangle of aimless thoughts. A mixture of love and of absurd sentiments was lifting her heart to the very heights of pleasure; until, suddenly, the chasm opened, and Laura flew with the sharpest of images back to yesteryear.

She looked down at her legs, the ones holding her up and she thought: What is that moving on the floor? Suddenly, she regained coherence and observed, with clarity, that the legs were hers, and then, she could not understand why she had been unable to identify them.

# VI

No. The school in the city was nothing like that place. They all bid her goodbye, her friends, the plants, the trees, and that road that took them to the top of the hill, where the school was.

Now... everything was so new... She could no longer talk with the animals, or the flowers, not even with the stones in the road. Her imagination was so great that entering this new world had left it in a weakened state, stifled by this world of paved streets, and buildings reaching up to the clouds, and that sticky, sour smell which she later learned was gasoline.

She remembered that puddle that she had admired so many times, watching those shapes with the bulky heads and dancing tails that never stopped moving transform into splendid frogs that croaked in the night.

But that puddle had also been left behind, and now she entertained herself by watching her new classmates.

Every day she arrived at home dying of sadness and with that heavy feeling in the pit of her stomach:

"Listen, Laura, you are important. You are a very bright girl, and you know very well that you are different, because you will reach great heights, darling. You are the queen of the castle... Can't you see we all think the same?"

"We all... And who is that...? Dad and you... I mean, do I have any brothers or sisters? I'm all alone, you know? A-lone."

At that, it seemed to Laura that she could see her mother's eyes fill with tears.

All of those memories came to Laura's mind with absolute clarity. Those little snippets of her childhood were burned upon her neurons. She remembered the gauze and Band-Aids on her knees, and the scars which would be visible forever, from the repeated falls off of the bike the Three Kings brought her one year. That was when she was nine years old.

"You still have one more wonderful present waiting for you, Laura. Look around and see if you can find it."

And then she went to work, running from one place to the other. "Cold, cold," they told her. And then, the moment arrived when her mother told her: "Warmer, *hot, hot...*" And before her there appeared a bicycle, hidden, leaning up against a post of the Hórreo[1], alongside the house...

From the vast window of her memory, Laura could smell, feel, watch, and admire... She would laugh and then feel overwhelmed... Today, behind the glass which separated her from the park, memories came back to her as she peeked through the cracks of that time past. Because then... was today. And today, where was today? What had she done this morning? Who was she now? Because her memories spoke of her, but... was it her? She was in the initial phase of Alzheimer's. The disease had already gotten to her.

Today, Laura was baffled by the swirls of words that would come and go as if they were ballroom dancers. With a cup of coffee in her hands, now cold, not yet touched by her lips, she was seated by the window... No, she was not looking at the park; she was still up in the

---

1 ˙N.B. – An *Hórreo* is a granary made of wood and resting on stone pillars, and is a common construction in Asturias.

branches of that tall tree with its wide crown, yearning for the freedom shared by those who could fly and make themselves comfortable on the highest branch of all the trees of the forest.

She would try to project her mind out over those things which in some way had marked her life, and then she would laugh or cry, depending on the moment she was living.

# VII

One never arrives at the whole truth, nor is one ever
kept completely apart from it.

**Aristotle**

Laura's story is subject to the ups and downs of life. There is nothing mysterious about it; we live out this earthly experience, we have our rocks and our asphalt; along the way we travel rocky roads and smooth roads. We think we are sunk forever and then, suddenly, one day, something makes us pull ourselves up once more. So, when there is a knock at our door, when someone makes us stop and reflect for a moment, we should realize that the question "Why me?" serves no purpose.

Many years after her separation, and shortly after she had celebrated her fiftieth birthday, marking the start of a new chapter for her... it was at that precise moment that she started feeling bad.

She had been quite stressed lately. As a result, she was sleeping only a few hours at a time – her normal response to stress. The school days were tiring her out, and one day she felt a sort of sharp pain in the side of her head. The pain grew stronger, until it began affecting her left eye. She felt dizzy.

"I feel awful. Do you mind getting someone to substitute my class? It's just that I am having trouble seeing, and my head hurts terribly ... I don't know... it's never happened to me before."

"No problem. Would you like us to accompany you?"

"No, it's not necessary. I'll take a taxi. I'm going to look for a neurologist in the medical directory, to have a look at me. That way at least, if it's not something in his area, he can tell me who I should see."

She made a call and they gave her an appointment for that same day.

The medical office was in downtown Gijón. Quite close to Paseo de Begoña.

The door to the building was locked, so she rang the bell. The door handle opened with a creak, and she entered the small vestibule leading to the stairwell. She felt cold, but it was not cold on the street. She noticed a closed-in, musty smell, the strong smell of dampness, and then she realized it was a smell she had never before experienced.

She went up. She had always been quite impatient, and now, of course, this was no time to be laid back. No.

She was anxious for them to rid her of this terrible pain...

A woman wearing a white coat met her at the door. She appeared to be a foreigner.

"Do you have an appointment, madam?"

"Yes. I called today, hoping the doctor would see me as soon as possible. I found him in the medical directory under neurologists. Really, the person who answered the phone was most generous. He gave me an appointment right away. I really appreciate it."

"Fine, wait here one moment, and I will show you in. Do you have insurance?"

"Yes," she said. And she showed her identification card as proof.

Laura took a seat. The waiting room had a bleak look about it. Antique furniture. The kind of furniture that provoked so much fear in her; what circumstances led to their inclusion in such a drab setting? She was alone. She felt even colder. The cold she felt came of loneliness.

How was it possible she had so little family? Only her father had a brother, the man who had graciously led her to the altar, and who had passed away leaving no children behind. She had no brothers or sisters, no cousins, no... just her daughter Ana, to whom she could not give any brothers or sisters, because her marriage had failed, and she had been left with no desire to ever start another relationship with anyone.

There were a few antique details which attracted her interest, but that was it. She preferred a light décor, as opposed to decoration that made use of dark colors or showy, wrought figures. On one wall, painted in ochre tones, there hung a few paintings, framed in ornate filigree.

Having heard "Come this way, please", she got up and followed to where the lady who opened the door for her was pointing.

"Ummmm, these symptoms may be hiding behind something else. Well, to be sure, I'll start from the beginning. Have you had any tests done recently?"

"No, the truth is I have always enjoyed very good health."

"Madam... how old did you say you were?"

"Fifty."

"If I may explain... we'll start with an MRI, and I'll do an in-depth study. I would like you to write a few pages relating what has been happening, whatever comes into your head. The tests will take us a few days."

"That's fine, but... is all this really necessary? The truth is, until this morning... I was fine. I just came in because my head hurts and I feel a little dizzy. That's all. Maybe I should have gone to see my family doctor, or... just taken a pain-reliever. The truth is, I just got nervous, and I don't know why I thought of a specialist... No, I don't think a study is called for. Certainly not."

"Yes... but things... sometimes things are more complex than they appear to be."

The following day, she took a simple aspirin, and the pain was gone. She almost decided not to go back for a diagnosis – she was not particularly interested. Her health had always been perfect, and she had never had any problem other than this one, which, in her opinion, was fleeting. Twenty days passed, and she received a phone call from the doctor's office telling her to come by and pick up the results.

She did not tell anybody anything... why worry her daughter, or her friends? No, it wasn't worth it.

After work let out, she went to her appointment.

The waiting room of the doctor's office was cold. Even colder than the last visit. There was a heavy energy in the air, weighing down on her heart. By the time the doctor arrived, she was having difficulty breathing. His face did not reflect even the smallest trace of tenderness. His hands, with their fat, stubby fingers and impeccable nails, gesticulated repeatedly, and his eyes did not meet hers. The white coat provided a particular professionalism, but the atmosphere remained heavy and the feeling of sadness continued to flood Laura's senses.

Laura stared at the floor and mused:

"It smells like sadness..."

"Excuse me, did I hear you correctly? Did you say it smells like sadness?"

"Oh! Don't mind me. It's a funny habit of mine. Ever since I was a little girl. I identify feelings and colors with smells. And I just felt a sharp pain in my stomach, and I perceive the smell of sadness."

"And what color is sadness?"

"It's brown."

"The truth is, you know, what you are saying is rather odd. I have never, in all my years in the profession, heard anything like it. By the way... have you come by yourself?"

"Yes. Is something wrong?"

"Well... I don't know how to tell you this."

"Whatever it is, tell me, do I have something serious?"

"It depends on how you look at it. You see... we have taken X-rays, an MRI, and countless other tests. We have detected a multitude of ischemias – anomalies, for a person of your age – as well as other alterations of the neurons. We have also detected beta-amyloid plaques. These plaques clump together and merge with other molecules, neurons and non-nerve cells; they are found in the hippocampus, a structure in the brain that helps to encode memories, thoughts and decision making..."

"And this means...?"

"Listen... and so you understand me, your brain is moth-eaten."

"Excuse me, you're telling me my brain is... moth-eat-en?"

"Not exactly, but we could qualify it as such, looking at the X-rays."

"Good God! This can't be. It can't be. It's... impossible," she laughed nervously. "I imagine that, for you to be able to tell me this, you must have sought professional confirmation, with other doctors... With... I don't know... I mean no offense. But, I think it is so shocking..., so shocking, that... I don't know..., it's hard to accept what you have said, and I imagine I won't be able to accept what you are telling me without going back and consulting with other professionals."

"I am sorry... you must come to terms with what is happening to you. You must take very good care of yourself. Don't drink alcohol, or smoke. Take long walks... It's important not to stress yourself out over anything."

"I'll have you know that the amount of alcohol I have consumed in my life wouldn't harm a baby. And I have never smoked. Stress, I've gone through stress. So, there, you are right."

"I am not saying that that has been the cause of your current situation. I am only advising you that, from now on, you must take care of yourself, and, I repeat, avoid stress. Also, you should know that neither your headache, for which you came to see me, nor the dizziness have had anything whatsoever to do with this disease. It was providential, your having come to see me. I know of one other case, just one, like yours. A woman in Luanco. That being said; please, do not stress yourself."

"Well... this is a fine moment not be stressed... And how long can I count on maintaining my mental faculties? According to you..."

"Okay, in five years – and it may be sooner – you will begin to lose your memories. Within five years more or less... you will no longer be yourself."

"How is that possible? I don't have any symptoms. I practice my profession without the slightest problem. I... have no cause to feel that something in my brain is not working properly."

"But, things are what they are. We will have to continue running tests and many, many treatments; though I can't assure you of anything."

And then, Laura, with a folder under her arm, stuffed with the medical tests they had just handed to her, headed down to the street. Her eyes were bulging, the sockets sunken in, her heart was palpitating, and a whole host of new sensations pressed hard against her temples. It couldn't be... that this sad disease, this thief of memories, would claim her.

She had so much to do. Her daughter, her history... all of it would go off to sleep in the hidden void into which everything disappears. It would be that black hole, destroyer, tireless friend to the enemy, dedicated to absorbing an entire life. A person's life turns out to be a difficult road on which to build experiences. A life belongs to the person who works at it one day after the other, and that the tangle of neurons that is our brain should fall asleep or cohabitate with injustice cannot be permitted.

Her work, her friends... her daughter. She could not stop being her and yet still be her. Because she would be like an empty shell. Like that cracked egg that liberates its contents. And those contents, where do they go? Down the drain of oblivion, where no one may receive what it took so much effort, so much work, so many sorrows and joys to build. Laura squeezed that rosary of litanies she leveled at herself, as she headed towards the parking garage.

Her blue car... that blue that smelled of home, of that twenty-seven of yesteryear, which once adorned the mill house. She stepped on the clutch, pressed down on the gas and headed towards the highway. One hundred thirty, one forty, one fifty... What did it matter! She wanted to die. She didn't want to be a burden, and she would never accept that who and what she was would be taken away from her. It doesn't matter if they take what you have, but what you are ... that belongs to you. You have cultivated it. You have worked it. You have lived it...

In the end, she was coherent once more, and she reduced her speed. She realized she had been playing not only with her life, but with the lives of others, and then a shiver ran the length of her spine. She didn't want to make it home. She took an exit on her right, and then, with her lights on she drove slowly in the direction of Campa de Torres. She parked the car and got out. It was cold, but she didn't care.

She walked towards the cliff, and the wind blew her skirt about, making the cold even colder than her loneliness. Colder even than those thoughts which lay within her heart. Colder than the smell of black, that faint smell of goodbye to life. It was dusk; she was breathing heavily, and her breathing propelled memories that penetrated her Soul: memories of her childhood, her home, her wonderful parents, the house on the Mill, the big house they lived in later on, full of light, on the side of the hill... memories of her beloved daughter, Ana... Ana, like her mother's name... and she held close each memory, each sweet moment. The loneliness pressed down hard on her chest, and she began to take off her jacket, then, quickly, her blouse, her skirt... She picked up all of her belongings and threw them over the side of the cliff, as a preamble to the act of throwing herself over. She was alone. No one else was around. She looked first to one side, then the other, and then started to run; gasping for breath and shouting, her words, portents: now it would be all over for her. She would not live to see herself end up a zombie, alive but not living.

She headed quickly to the car. She tried to leave something in writing for her daughter, Ana; so that, when they found what traces were left behind of her departure, she would understand that her sudden departure had not been for nothing. She would understand that he mother did not know how to face that life that someone else had scripted for her, and that she wasn't capable of facing her empty destiny.

She looked anxiously for a pen in her bag, which lay on the seat next to her. A piece of paper... where the hell was the paper? The datebook she always carried with her was nowhere to be found. She opened the envelope containing that horrible diagnosis and then... then... a soft music seemed to reach her ears, and the blue lettering of the doctor's name, written on the cardboard flap, it smelled of home to her. It enveloped her in the scent of family, and then, something seized her hands and gripped her heart.

Ana... my dearest Ana. I can't leave you. What am I going to do? What was I about to do? God! I can't abandon you. She broke down and cried, everything became blurry; her lost eyes could just make out the lights of a few ships on their way from the Port. But what mattered to her was not the goodbye to life. She was prepared to give up her life a thousand times over, so long as the end for her would be a physical end. She wanted to be in the position to say that it was all over, completely, rather than having a piece of herself, her very self, disappear while leaving the rest of her behind.

And the abyss, the rock strewn coast down below her, invited her to jump, again and again. She studied her arms; in the shadows they appeared as wings to her. She glanced down at her legs, and they looked like two timid brushstrokes resting upon heavy blocks of sand and floating above a narrow void. She regained her wits and, staring at the ground, realized that she had thrown up. It was then that a feeling of panic washed over her. She thought again of her daughter, and of what was to become of her. She hadn't been able to give her any brothers or sisters because she hadn't had time; because Ana's father ran off with another woman, because she never loved anyone again, because everything shut tight after that sad and agonizing separation.

And she thought again of everything around her, of her friends, her students, and then she ran to her vehicle, which had remained there, waiting for her. Once more safely inside, she slipped down the highway, towards her home, without any clothes on.

On the way home, she thought: I'll enter through the garage, and I'll take the elevator up. Heaven, keep me from being seen half naked by anyone...

She had no problems arriving home, and no one saw her. She put away all the papers she had been carrying. She got in the shower and scrubbed her body, vigorously, in a rage, consciously trying to hurt herself, rebellious in attitude.

The scouring she gave herself seemed to calm her down, and she dried herself off, a little at a time. She put on moisturizing cream, and after, a pink dress. She suddenly remembered the tangled tufts of sugar of that same color that they always used to buy, every Sunday, from the lady with the Percheron horse who passed in front of the house. And then, a hint of sweetness invaded her.

She waited patiently for her daughter to arrive. On the small living room table she placed a fine tablecloth with embroidered edges. White. Suddenly, she remembered that dark Church that, on so many

Sundays, she had visited as a young girl. A shiver raced through her body, and she perceived that almost forgotten smell, of white.

She went to the china cabinet and took down two cups of cut Bohemian glass from the glassware set she so rarely used. She only put it out on special occasions, and there had been few of those in her lifetime, because she had had little to celebrate. She placed them one in front of the other, delicately and with great care, and then, she opened a bottle of Rioja. Red. She removed the cork, so as to allow the contents of the bottle to breathe. Someone had once explained to her that a good wine should be left uncorked once it has been opened.

She prepared a tray of thinly sliced ham and pork loin, and a little cheese.

She remembered the silver cutlery that for some time now had remained in the silverware drawer, and she also brought out the small bread dish, complemented elegantly by a cloth trimmed with festoons, upon which she carefully placed a small piece of bread that she had softened in the microwave.

She turned on the television, dried her tears, and waited for her daughter.

Her daughter... her whole life... that was what she meant to her. She had had her when she was twenty-five. The best thing to ever happen to her, she had always thought.

She had green eyes, like her grandfather and like herself, but darker. Her complexion was dark, perhaps in memory of a long forgotten ancestor. She was always a *delight*.

"It's a shame your grandmother and your grandfather didn't get to know you, sweetheart!" she used to tell her.

"I have other grandparents too, Mom. And they love me a lot. Now, I know they blame you for the separation, and that they don't love you, but they do love me," her daughter had told her one time, and this was the reason those persons no longer existed for her... Blame her for a separation, when the only thing she had done was uncover the deceitfulness of the man who was once her husband?

Even though they had separated when their daughter was still little, once upon a time she and Arturo had maintained a pleasant relationship. He would pick their daughter up each weekend, and he visited her as often as he wished, until he apparently found another true love and remarried, once the divorce had been finalized; Laura had conceded the divorce without asking for any explanation. She made a point of finding out the name of his new wife; but it wasn't Monica. That was the romance that had succeeded in ending their marriage. He had had two more children, and it made Laura happy to know that her daughter had brothers. Only in this way would Ana not feel alone, and so Laura continued to encourage Ana's relationship with her father's family, for the good of her daughter.

Ana had studied Journalism. She had lived in Madrid for four years, and afterwards she returned to Asturias, to work as an editor in a local newspaper. She worked long hours, but her job was fulfilling, and it made her happy.

And immersed in these thoughts which helped to drive away the sadness left by the heavy blow she had received, Ana arrived home.

She remained seated while the joyful young woman kissed her and then remarked on how strange it was to see those glasses out, and that wine and the silverware ... and...

The two of them sat for a while and drank a toast, and then:

"Mom, you seem sad. How was your day?"

"The usual. Fine."

"Well, you seem a bit down. Is something wrong?"

"No. It's just, you see... let me tell you... I hadn't planned to say anything to you, sweetheart, but you know... I am such a bigmouth... and if I don't tell you, what am I going to do? Who is going to understand me better than you?

You see..."

It was a long conversation; the words followed one after the other, and then the tears and the feelings of emptiness ...

"Don't pay it any mind. Tomorrow we'll look for solutions. I don't have any faith in this doctor, not in his tests... none of it. You'll go to a hospital where they can do a proper study. And whatever else is necessary. If we have to travel across all of Spain, all of the world, we will do it! But I am not going to leave you in the hands of some 'quack'."

A few days later, they already had a number of appointments for Laura to have an exhaustive examination done.

After a thousand tests of every type, more questions, and many more answers, she was told:

"Listen... the diagnosis they gave you, and with all due respect from our team – the team which has studied you – of course is unfounded. There is no basis for telling you your brain is moth-eaten. We have never heard that term used. The headache and the dizziness that led you to seek out that initial consultation have nothing to do with what was detected in the later studies. However, there is something. It is true that an anomaly shows in the tests. Really, there is nothing concrete that indicates to us that you are going to suffer a degenerative disease, or that you are going to suffer from Alzheimer's. Certainly, the tests do suggest you are suffering an alteration. We cannot say for certain whether you will suffer from the disease, or whether it will be relatively soon, later, or perhaps never. Who knows what turn these things might take! Regarding some aspects, we don't wish to call into question the diagnosis they have given you, and, certainly, we should not rule out the possibility that it points to an alteration. But today, still, there is no solution to that terrible disease, and so, even if the results were clearly positive, there would be no adequate drug available to us, nor any vaccine to eliminate the process.

With a pharmacological treatment, all we would be doing is slowing the disease down, but there is no cure. And so, do you really wish to know whether you will suffer from Alzheimer's within a short – or even shorter – period of time? Or from any other disease which might cause you to lose your memories?"

All of the silence... all the silence that could possibly be heard... was heard within that very silence, until finally:

"No. I don't want to know."

And with that, the door closed with a loud thud, much like the sound made by the beating of Laura's heart.

# VIII

Time is nothing more than the space between
our memories.

Henri Frédéric Amiel

A number of months had passed since that first time she was twirling her fork without knowing what it was. Laura was still leading what seemed to be her normal life. They prescribed Arizept, a pill which they said might slow down the process of the disease. She would still go to the store, pulling her shopping cart along, but now she would leave the house accompanied by certain obsessions.

She was obsessed with the possibility of casually running into someone she knew and having to converse with them. Because she was aware that she often couldn't find the right words. Sometimes, she would say things she didn't mean to say, and then she would feel ashamed.

One day, she asked her daughter, "What is happening to me?" Only to later forget she had asked that question, because her life had once again assumed complete normality.

But then, suddenly, she would utter a phrase that no one could understand and then repeat it again and again. She felt threatened by passersby in the street, or by people conversing in front of the building, or by folks who entered her home. She was totally helpless and vulnerable.

She would go out, and, sometimes, her life went on as it always had. And then, without warning, she would feel an intense sadness pressing upon her stomach, and she would find herself surrounded by potential enemies.

She would race back home, seeking refuge; but in a little while, the uncertainty would return, and she would find herself in a strange place, unable to recognize her own home. Then, once again, normality would return and leave her with her heart still thumping.

"Ana, give me a *susuli.*"

"What is it you want, Mom? Tell me clearly, you know how."

And Laura would hold out her hand for a newspaper that for days had been among a stack of magazines and other newspapers from weeks past.

Ana was losing heart as time went on. Her mother was no longer the person she once was.

Sometime they let her dress herself, and... she would put on two or three layers of clothing. Or she would put on her coat, even though she was not going to leave the house.

She continued to experience mood swings, and, fairly often, she would curse; until then, no one could ever remember hearing her swear.

She became more difficult to deal with, and one day... many months later...

"How are you, Mom? Have you had a good day?"

"Mom? Did you call me Mom?" She smiled, and then she burst out laughing. "Do you really think I'm your mother?"

"Mama... are you kidding? It's me, Ana. Your daughter, A–na."

"I'm sorry, Miss, but I am not your mother. I've never had any children."

And right then, Ana felt like an orphan; she felt dead. She could feel the beating of her heart and a huge knot in her throat, and it squeezed her so tightly, as if, suddenly her body hurt with the pain of this scene, which she could never forget; she felt as if an assassin had arrived to cut her throat from ear to ear.

Cringing, shaking, bawling, she made her way to the bathroom. She couldn't breathe. She brought her hands down to her sides and then, without knowing what she was doing, she opened the faucet and stuck her head under the stream of cold water.

For a moment, she was absolutely beside herself with grief. She tried breathing deeply, and then, she heard a voice from the back of the house, by the large window, saying:

"Sweetheart, are you home already?"

Ana endured sad ups and downs, from one day to the next. She recalled that day when her mother informed her of the sentence fate had passed upon her, and she also remembered the deal they had made at that moment. Her mother had asked her to study her eyes, to look beyond her gaze, when she was convinced that she was no longer coherent. But today, it is still too soon, Ana thought.

All was not lost, because many times that was still her, the lapses were only occasional, and she was still able to lead a normal life; she was still capable of asking for what she wanted, even if she might call it by a different name.

Laura was experiencing many moments where she would remain silent, though she would move her lips. No. She was not praying, as her daughter had at first concluded. She was simply moving her lips.

"Mom, for God's sake what are you doing following me around with a raised mop? Do you plan to hit me with a mop? Why do you have your lips pressed together so tightly like that? And those eyes ... God, Mom, your eyes are popping out of your head..."

"Witch! You... are a witch – you are wicked. Out of my house!"

"Mom, it's me! Can't you see me, Mom? Can't you see I'm taking care of you as much as my job will allow, I'm by your side as much time as I can be? It's me, Mom! Mom...it's me!"

Once the uproar had died down, a short time later, Helena arrived. She had finally started working full time. She was looking after Ana's mother, and this was why Ana had decided not to send her mother to an adult daycare center, something she had considered sometime ago.

Helena hugged the young woman who was sobbing, howling... she tried to comfort this young woman who was frightened to death and who for years had been aware of her mother's sentence.

It was overwhelming her; costing her very life. Her heart was so heavy... she never would have imagined this situation, so much loneliness and so much sadness at once.

"Mom, why do you want so many tomatoes?"

"I don't know, baby. I bought them this morning; the truth is, I can't figure out why I bought nothing but tomatoes. And, what's more... we don't eat them often. We don't like them very much, remember? I didn't even get bread! I'm sorry... I guess it slipped my mind."

"You know something, daughter? I think Aurora, the neighbor in 1-B, the one who has that notions shop, I think she wants to steal my purse. She's always looking at my handbag, and sometimes I see her spying on me out of the corner of her eye."

"Mom, come off it, for God's sake, don't think strange things, you can trust her. Can't you see she has lived next door all her life?"

"Yes, I know that, but her intentions are bad ... I have seen it in her look, and I also have to tell you how ..."

"Don't make me laugh, Mom, I don't want to hear any more nonsense, you understand?"

"You know what I think? Maybe you are in cahoots with her and... well, I guess you won't believe me either when I tell you that the other day, when I was walking down the street, a man was following me. He was attractive, tall, with gray hair, and he winked at me. I think he's looking to get something going with me, but don't think for a moment that I am going to fall into his arms, I'm stronger than that, and I will not give any other man the chance. And do you know who it is I am talking about? None other than Joaquín, the husband of Doña Teresa, the tobacconist. If I were ever to say anything..."

"Mom, that's impossible, that gentleman was just operated on for his prostrate, and he's got enough on his hands just trying to survive..."

"Yeah, yeah... What would you know?"

"By the way, Mom... don't take this the wrong way, but Helena tells me that lately you are leaving your underwear on the bathroom floor, and also that when you shower you leave a big puddle on the floor. I don't want to reproach you for anything, but I would expect you to understand that the poor lady shouldn't have to go around picking up... well, you understand me."

"Understand you? Not at all. What she's saying isn't true... How could you believe your mother is capable of doing something like that? When have I ever left the bathroom looking like I had been in it? Tell me... when?"

"That is why I found it so strange. And that is why I am letting you know..."

"By the way, baby... I have had a fight."

"A fight? For God's sake, Mother... a fight with whom?"

"With our neighbor next door, because yesterday I turned the television on, and do you know what she did? Well, a ton of frogs poured out and got through the whole house. And while I was picking one up here and another there, I could hear her door closing.

Since there was no way to put them all back in the television, I ran to her door, and I told her off – she had it coming. I let her have it, because she is really disagreeable. Dis-a-gree-able. And I've known that for a long time, I just didn't want to say anything."

"But, Mom. You have always been so restrained. You have always been a very coherent person, and now it turns out, you think the whole world is against you. It's not true. It's your imagination. Ignore those ravings and consider yourself happy. Think yourself happy and you will be happy, Mother."

"Why are you calling me 'Mother'? You never did before."

"I don't know. Maybe I'm raving too. Oh, Mom, this situation is so difficult!"

After that day, Ana could still hold short conversations with her mother once in a while, and they would even laugh together, making plans or discussing situations from the past.

Today, in the immense window looking out over the Park in front of her, with her legs crossed, she continued living, as that plant in the garden can live, or that stone in the river, often talking as if nothing were happening to her. Completely normal.

# IX

"You have gotten good grades, and we are very happy with you, honey. You will be a great person. You are a very sharp young girl, but what we are going to ask of you, is that you keep your feet on the ground. Don't start telling stories that live only in your imagination. Sweetheart, try to be more serious – you are eleven years old, and that's old enough to know that people might not think you are in your right mind if you go around saying that each color has its own scent, and whatever other stories of yours that live in the world of fantasy. Please, daughter, be coherent."

"Okay. What does it mean to be coherent?"

"It means be sensible, sweetie. Be sensible. Use sense and good judgment. Leave the world of fantasy behind."

"Alright."

"This year they have changed the school uniform. You will be wearing a gray tartan, and you will have a hat with a ribbon. Those are the rules."

"There is no way! A hat with a ribbon... Mom, that's outrageous – all the girls are going to look at me and laugh! It was bad enough that day with the diadem and the flowers."

"I repeat... that's the way it is, end of story."

"Okay, are you sure we will all be dressed the same?"

"Of course you will."

Time went by, and at thirteen she became a woman. And as surely as this event marks the life of every girl who enters into adolescence around the world, this event marked Laura.

"Daughter, it's nothing. It's just that... you have become a woman. You're thirteen now! Don't worry. But you'll have to take special care of yourself. You have entered your fertile period, and it can lead into trouble... you understand. You've got to be sensible."

"Mom... it's just that, the girls at school, well, sometimes we talk about it, but until now you've never said anything to me about it. That's why I thought that, maybe, it would not be right. I don't know... I mean something I shouldn't talk about. But, Mom, it's just... it's a pain. What makes you think I'm going to... Oh, brother! What a pain. Fertile; that word makes me think of Daddy's garden."

When she returned to school, the next day, she made it known between whispers that she had crossed to the other side. She was no longer a girl. She was already preparing herself for when she would be able to show off her chest.

When she turned fifteen... she fell in love. Her first love.

There were no dates, not even a kiss, not even the brush of her leg against his, but she dreamed night and day, and when she woke up in the morning, she did so having dreamed of a sweet kiss.

He was a football player on the local team. The manner in which he followed her to school in his car was curious, driving and talking all the while with her, since of course she hadn't wanted to get in with him. After all, that kind of thing was frowned upon, and her parents might find out, and... He drove slowly, alongside Laura, because in those times, there were almost no cars on the roads, and those that were on the road had the blessings of the neighbors.

Dreaming... dreaming was her best subject. She had strong ideas, and she defended her theories stubbornly, though often enough she used reasoning to do so. She was shy, and her shyness prevented her from speaking. She would feel as if a strong pressure was tightening around her throat. But, sometimes, when she couldn't stand it anymore...

"Cristina's little brother has died. Poor little thing! He wasn't baptized yet and he will remain in limbo," Sister Pilar was saying, a sorrowful look on her face.

"What? What do you mean he will remain in limbo? That can't be! If God is just and good, He can't do that."

"Do you realize what you are saying, Laura? Such fallacy! How could you dare to you say something so horrible? I cannot believe it... what you need to do, first of all, is leave the classroom, and the Mother Superior will have a talk with you later. Such an aberration coming from the mouth of a little brat. And go confess! I suppose you didn't go far enough a few months ago when you said that Eternal Hell didn't exist? Hmm? The reprimand you received wasn't enough to make you change your opinion?"

"Excuse me, Sister, but Eternal Hell cannot exist either; if God is just and good, He can't do that with a human being, even if we are not as perfect as He expected us to be."

"Get out of here! We will have a talk with your parents. These are grounds for expulsion. Don't forget that you are attending a Catholic, religious school."

And the reprimand was so serious that Laura was punished for a long time and was not allowed to go to the cinema on Saturdays.

She was a difficult case, her parents said, and they were constantly worrying about where being a bigmouth might lead her.

And Saturday was that magical day when she didn't have to wear her uniform. Her Saturday dress was something special, and her Sunday dress to go to Mass was even more special.

At fifteen, of course, she didn't wear her hair in pigtails anymore, and the ribbons which once adorned them were put away in a drawer of old memories.

The stairs out of the house were witness to how she would roll her skirt up under her waistline, so that the *bunched up* material became, by work and grace, a miniskirt. Of course, nice girls were forbidden to wear miniskirts, but she was resourceful and used this trick to shorten her skirt by a few centimeters. Later, when she arrived back home, in the same spot, she would roll the skirt back down. That left the skirt a bit mashed up and wrinkled, but that was not important once the goal had been achieved.

"Where are you coming back from, dear?"

"From the cinema, Mom."

"What did you see?"

"'An angel has arrived', with Marisol."

"Did you like it?"

"Yes. A lot. Well, good night, I am going to bed, I am not hungry, and anyway we ate sunflower seeds and tiger nuts."

"Next time don't do that; it's essential that you eat dinner in order to do well at school. Sweetheart, you know, you are at a bad age, you're growing very quickly, and you need nourishment. Make sure that's the last time."

Then Laura went to her room and daydreamed about how she had danced all evening, with the boy of her dreams. She had really gone to a party, but, because she was as sweet as honey, as soft as velvet, and looked as if she had never broken a plate, there was no reason for her parents to doubt her word.

The posters they hung at the entrance to the cinema itself, with sequences of the film, were interpreted by Laura in her own way, and with the conviction of her tireless imagination, everything was believable. No one would ever have guessed that really she had not sat for two hours, watching Marisol, the star of those popular films.

The wholesome practices of that time set the limits, and the litany they were always feeding you was repeated a thousand times over...

"Be careful, boys sometimes look to spend time with girls that are easy. And you, you have to set the limits. Don't let him rub his body against yours when you dance. I know, you're still too young, but I mean when you start going out dancing."

"I know how to take care of myself. Don't worry."

"You know how to defend yourself? That is naïve on your part. You always think the best of everyone. Believe me, things are not as you think. "Also... don't forget: never get into a stranger's car. He can take you off to some field somewhere and force himself on you..."

"Oh, come on... force himself on me! What you are saying is such nonsense!"

"Listen, what I said. You just study, and don't do anything foolish. Otherwise, you might send your father and me to an early grave."

Rules and rules and more rules, really, who could have created so much artifice? Why can't I hug who I like if I like him?

Los Brincos, Fórmula V, los Bravos, the Beatles, and so many other groups whose music inspired her to dream and helped free her from the monotony of her classes, like when they would sing 'Alouette' in that French class that never seemed to end:

«Alouette, gentille alouette,

Alouette, je te plumerai.

Je te plumerai la tête.

Je te plumerai la tête.

Et la tête ! Et la tête !

Alouette, Alouette !

And between 'Alouette', los Brincos and the Beatles, Karina, Adamo and many others who helped define her schooldays, the end of the school year arrived. The pre-university studies were about to end, and her eyes were set on the University.

The truth is that Laura, felt appreciation, from the bottom of her heart, for the teachings the religious order had given her, but, at the same time, she couldn't help thinking that many of the Religion lessons made no sense at all. Obviously. They were nonsense and collapsed under their own weight. They were stories, which often no one could believe.

"Dear students: You must always remember, each and every day of your lives, these teachings we have given you. Don't forget that each one of you is a reflection in which a part of society sees itself, and you must teach by your example, beautiful and tolerant.

You must carry the word of God with you, wherever you may go, and know that people are human beings. Do not make distinctions between one class and another, and realize that you are Catholics, and that your duty is to continue the work with which we have entrusted you, pursuing eternal salvation. Remember that good deeds shall be rewarded and bad deeds shall be punished."

"Only Catholics can save themselves? This is a litany I have always heard, and which I do not share. Really, only Catholics can save themselves?"

"That is so, Laura. Thus it is written."

"But... if someone hasn't had the chance to be Catholic, what happens?"

"He will not attain eternal salvation, because he has not been baptized, nor has he performed the rest of the sacraments necessary to get to eternal Heaven."

"Well, it's not fair. I don't see it that way. I believe creed doesn't matter – what matters are the positive and negative experiences each one of us has lived. Even the negative, one can learn from it, without being denied entrance into the Heavenly Kingdom."

"Miss Laura. I believe what you have just said is utter foolishness. In all the time you have been at this school, since the very day you arrived – I think you were ten years old – until now, when you are eighteen, your questions have verged on insolence. Personally, I think you haven't learned anything in all that time. Not only that, but you have also been a bad influence for some of the students who have heard you speak. I am very sorry. I think you are moving too far away from the divine commandments, and this will lead to serious problems for you throughout your life."

"Maybe you are right. I have learned a lot with you during these years. But something tells me that it is possible for things to be gray. Not just black or white. One thing is the rectitude and good deeds of the individual, and another thing, a quite different thing, is the lack of tolerance on the part of religion. That's all."

"Take a seat, and I hope you have life full of successes, and may God never leave your side!"

# X

**Do not concern yourself with making your face beautiful, but instead concentrate on adorning the Soul, with honorable studies.**

*Thales of Miletus*

"His Excellency, The Head of the Spanish State, and in his name the Minister of Education and Science, in recognition of the satisfactory completion of the course prescribed by the faculty of the University of Oviedo, in accordance with the applicable provisions and circumstances, by Miss Laura Rodríguez de las Heras, born November 7, 1953, confers this Degree of Bachelor of Arts in Philsophy and Letters, on January 25, 1976, with HONORS.

This degree grants the holder the right to practice the profession and to enjoy all the rights, privileges and honors prescribed by the applicable provisions and circumstances."

Helena had been asked to repeat phrases and songs to her mother... and to get her to look at herself in the mirror; but now... she no longer recognized herself.

Laura stuttered and was unable to utter more than a few sentences at a time, and she appeared to have grown shy. Nonetheless, each time her daughter came home, or her friends, or Helena, arrived at the house, she would ask them for a kiss. When they planted a kiss on her cheek, she would give a big smile.

She loved to receive cuddles and caresses, and she would show it by closing her eyes tighter and tighter, as if she wanted to reveal all the love she had inside, but didn't know how.

Laura paced up and back, as if she were an animal in a cage. When asked her date of birth, her age, her first and last names, she would sometimes answer correctly and then smile, waiting for approbation, and other times... other times... she had no idea who she was, never mind the date and place in which she had come into the world.

Ana had become like the Guadiana River[2] for her mother – now you see her, now you don't. Sometimes Ana was a stranger to her, and then, her daughter would cry and run off to her room, while her mother remained behind, looking on but understanding nothing of what had happened. At another moment, she would once again be recognized as Ana. Her Ana, whom she had always known.

Lately, Laura was given to recite all the rivers of Europe from memory. She would not miss a single one, although along with some of the names she would include incoherent words. At other times, she would start off with the Greek alphabet, reciting from alpha to omega without stuttering a bit.

Sometimes, she would not make it to the bathroom in time, and she would wet herself. Then, she would watch the liquid spills out, while she parted her legs. She would remain still, without knowing what to do. She didn't understand what was happening to her. Other times, she wouldn't care, but most times, she would open her eyes wide, and her mouth... the smile of a helpless little girl. She was navigating between the reality of the situation and the real situation. Perhaps she observed, for tenths of a second at a time, that she was not in her right mind, but at the same time, she had forgotten what it was to be in one's right mind...

---

2 ˙ N.B. – Controversy has always surrounded the source of the Guadiana River. Comparing a person or thing to the Guadiana suggests that their comings and goings are unpredictable.

Her eyes cast about a threatening look as she slowly walked over to the side of the window.

Today, the sky was very blue, and the birds were darting about. The news on television had said that viewers would soon note the drops in temperatures, and so Laura, with the heat on, sat in the armchair in which she felt most comfortable.

She continued to go out in the company of Helena, or with her daughter when her job permitted.

At home, she liked to take apples out of one basket and place them in another. When she finished her 'work', she would smile so as to receive approval for her efforts, and after a short time, she would begin to return the fruit to where it first came from. She was capable of spending an entire morning like that.

A number of folks had told Ana that it would be a good thing to get her a little dog, because sometimes a strong current of affection develops between the human being and the animal. But... it didn't turn out that way.

One afternoon, some months back, Helena arrived with a Golden Retriever puppy. Small, blond and playful. She put the well-groomed puppy in Laura's lap, and her mother began to cry, saying, "Troski! Troski! I want Troski... this isn't my dog..." And so, the animal was returned to where it first came from.

Today was the day when she had to go for another checkup, to observe the progress of what had already become a harsh sentence.

"What is your name? What is your age? Where were you born? What are your parents' names? Are you single? How many children do you have? What year were you born? Do you have brothers or sisters? And now, repeat in the same order: 'house', 'fruit', 'milk', 'day'..."

Now... nothing. A few right answers, by chance. But... now the deterioration was more than palpable. The first time she had come, she had gotten almost all the questions right, but today...

That time they had prescribed a treatment to slow down the advance of the inevitable; they prescribed it to her when she spoke of her obsessions, of her fear that friends, or her own family, were going to steal her purse. Or of her fear of fear itself. Or of often having to face a terrifying loneliness, even when in the company of others.

Then, the doctor took Ana aside and told her:

"Listen... it would be better if we began to use the medication more intensely. The truth is that she is heading where I said she would be, but... it can be slowed down, and her quality of life will not deteriorate in a short space of time, although, as you know quite well, when Alzheimer's comes at such an early age, everything goes much more quickly. At this age the illness is much more severe. I am very sorry about everything that is happening. It is a constant I see here every day. The truth is that, people are living longer, and over time, the disease develops frequently enough. But cases like your mother's – she is still young – well, we do not often see them. We do know that her life will be shortened."

"So... In your opinion, how long will she live?"

"I can't tell you anything. Simply, you should be prepared. It's a very hard road for her and, of course, for her caretakers."

"We have a person we trust completely who is with her all day. I am an only child, and I work a full time schedule. I cannot do much more, but... I hope to always be at her side... By the way... could this disease have anything to do with emotionally upsetting events? You see, my mother, she lost her father and her mother at almost the same time. And her marriage with my father... well, you understand what I mean..."

"No. We believe that has nothing to do with it. Does she exhibit any aggressive behavior?"

"Sometimes. A few days ago, she was with Helena, the lady who takes care of her. They were taking a relaxing stroll. My mother was carrying an umbrella, and without saying a word, when they passed by this one woman, she hit her with all her might, and that is quite a lot… as I was saying, she gave her a tremendous shot with the umbrella. She is unpredictable. Other times, she wants to hit me. She gets easily offended and swears – something I never heard her do until she became ill."

"Try to take things calmly. The deterioration will come, and there is nothing that can be done about it."

Laura, until quite recently, remembered that heavy blow, when she was in her second year at the university, and her father died of a heart attack.

She had gotten off the bus and was walking down the street with some classmates. Turning the corner, she observed a tumult of people and an ambulance in front of her apartment building.

A violent shudder swept through her, and, without uttering a word, she took off running until …

"Move back, please. Leave the doorway free – they have to come down with the stretcher…"

"A stretcher!! Where are they bringing a stretcher down from?"

"Please, move to the side. Wait, I can't let you by…"

But Laura could tell that whoever it was they were bringing down in the stretcher, was family. She knew this because she could hear that they were not coming down from the first floor, or the second, but rather, the third floor.

She had known something was going on in her house, from the moment she turned the corner. She tried to go up the stairs, someone told her to stop, and a neighbor ran up and gathered her up in her arms. At that moment, there was no longer any doubt, and she asked, "My father? My mother? What happened? What happened?"

And shortly after, the stretcher came down, accompanied by four people, and behind them her mother, crying and clutching at Laura.

There were almost no questions asked; the two women wept. They wept as they would weep during the rest of the time that life would allow them to be together.

They were never able to determine how this could happen to a person so young, in such good shape, without an ounce of fat on him and whose habits were healthy.

The loss was so tremendous that, from that very moment on, his wife stopped living. The love between them had always been obvious. Sometimes they argued, but rarely did they stay mad long. And so, her mother's grief weighed heavy, and she no longer felt any joy in living. Not even her darling Laura could do anything to help her to once more be the person she had been.

And Laura completed her university studies and began to work as a high school teacher.

In those days, premarital relations were frowned upon, and maybe for that reason... their courtship was short.

They met one spring afternoon on Calle Corrida. There, on the street, a mutual friend introduced them to one another, and in that moment, Laura fell head over heels in love with Arturo, and, of course, Arturo fell just as hard for Laura.

Laura arrived to the church on the arm of her Uncle Pascual, with tears in her eyes, for her loving father, who had left so suddenly.

As they came out of the temple there were joyful hugs and rice everywhere, and a strong breeze which obligated the guests to seek shelter on the bus which would soon take them to the banquet.

The tables were distributed in a round shape, like a great Coliseum, set up so that the bride and groom, in the center, could be seen by everyone and participate and share the food and the happiness which filled the air.

A simple floral arrangement reigned majestic on top of each immaculately white tablecloth. The china was of the same pristine color, with gilded edges, which, along with the silver flatware, regal and heavy, made for a harmonious and elegant ensemble. The four crystal glasses and the small silver bread plate laid out with each service took up a large part of the table.

At that center table was Laura, radiant in white, with her hair put up in a bun, the style of which was inspired by Audrey Hepburn's in the film "Breakfast at Tiffany's". From her hair hung a long embroidered veil, with gilded edges of fine blonde lace. Arturo was at her side, wearing a dark suit and a carnation in his lapel, beaming with joy. He could not keep himself from gazing upon his love, who, after today, was finally his. Uncle Pascual and Ana were seated on the side of the bride, and Fidel and Antonia, the groom's parents, were next to her darling Arturo.

In the background, a piano played classical pieces, and with each morsel of food, the soul would swell with pleasure along with the stomach.

The pearl earrings, a gift from her mother, complemented her ears, and the day smelled red. To Laura the day smelled red; as red as the explosive carnations which used to dance to the sound of the wind upon the windows of that grand house when it was new, long ago; even today, she could recall their stays in that house, happy and so full of light. And did that blue scent reach her, the scent which for her meant home and family? No. The scent she took in, today, was red.

On the ring finger of her left hand, a diamond. Naked, unadorned. On the ring finger of her right hand, the wedding band. Sparkling golden, with letters and the date engraved on its inner face.

I will never take it off, she thought, as she furtively kissed her resplendent husband and rested her leg, affectionately on his, under the table.

Her imperial cut dress highlighted that slim, sculpted body, eliciting Arturo's comment: "You look so pretty, my love."

Her slender, stiletto heel shoes – as white as the dress itself – lay by her feet. Like this... slyly... the act going unnoticed by the rest of the guests.

"We wish you all the happiness in the world..." the guests would come up and say, while the newlyweds hugged all those wishing them eternal love.

There were toasts: one for the godparents, another for the parents, then for the friends, the guests, and, finally... the first dance as a married couple.

A chorus of voices hummed along as the young lovers danced a waltz, gliding across the dance floor.

The two hundred guests filled the room and a "Long live the newly-weds!" was heard again and again.

Arturo was a love. That is what everyone who knew him was saying, and Laura as well; after all, he really was her love. Her true love and, perhaps... her only one. No one else would ever captivate her heart, she mused, as she floated along to the rhythm of the waltz, in that elegant room in the restaurant on the outskirts of the city, the same day the 'I do' was heard in the Church of San Pedro.

They traveled all over Spain, from the North to the South, celebrating their honeymoon. In between stops they gave free reign to their love and to the physical contact which, now, was no longer sinful. They no longer had to avoid living that consuming passion, now that they had sworn their love before God, to love forever and ever.

# XI

**He who gets into brambles and into love will enter**
**when he wishes but not get out when he likes.**

**Plutarch**

"Mom, you look so thin... is something wrong? Are you feeling ill?"

"Sweetheart, my nerves are shot, and I was so busy preparing your wedding and all that I stopped eating. That's all..."

But really, she was not at all well, and when she could feel it in her bones, she decided that it was time to visit the doctor. Laura knew perfectly well that her mother, though she was aware of what was happening to her, had waited so as not to alarm anyone. That was the kind of person she was.

And then, one winter's day, her mother, the woman who had given her so much, ceased to exist. She left this life, quietly, without saying anything, dealing with her disease discreetly, just as she had dealt with everything all during her life. Laura did not wish, today, to remember those last days of her mother's life. They were the most painful days of her life, ending with the burial on a rain-soaked day... However, a short two months later, Ana was born. Ana, her only daughter.

The days went by and then, on Ana's second birthday, Arturo, arrived late.

It wasn't the first time he had come home late, but, on that day, precisely that day, it was unacceptable. So, when he came into the living room of their home, apologizing and smelling of perfume that was not hers, the expression on Laura's face changed.

And with each day, she clearly observed the way in which her husband was acting more and more distant. The mechanical kiss when he arrived home, and then:

"Is something wrong? You seem so strange, with each day that goes by... a little more, Arturo. Did I do something to you that you didn't like?"

"No, there's nothing wrong with me, and you haven't done anything to me that I didn't like. Look... I'm getting a little tired of all this foolishness. It's always the same with you. You're becoming hysterical."

"No. That's not true. I am not becoming hysterical – simply... you don't tell me you love me anymore, and you're not showing interest in things the way you used to, until not so long ago. The truth is that in the last six months, you're not the same."

"Right... now comes the litany of complaints... And you? I suppose you are showing interest in me? You're always reproaching me when you should be reproaching yourself."

The family environment was becoming tenser with each passing day. The quiet spaces, the spaces of quiet words were a constant.

The house in which they lived was large and full of light and offered views of a beautiful park. And it had enough empty spaces for them to be apart from one another and never even touch each other.

There were separate beds, and many tears rolled down the sides of Laura's pillow:

"I would like to know what has happened to us. I want to fix our relationship, Arturo... I'd like to do it for our little girl and for us. Look around... we have everything we could want – we could be happy, like in the beginning."

"Consider the fact that, perhaps, this has been your fault, and later we'll talk. I am fed up... fed up with so much blame placed on me. And you? Think carefully about whether you haven't changed since the moment the girl was born. No. It's not that I've been pushed into the background; it's that I don't even exist for you anymore.

"Don't blame me again, and return to our bedroom if you want. It was you who decided to sleep in another room, so... stop and look at what you are doing, because I... I don't plan to put up with this situation any longer..."

Then Laura considered the possibility that she had been intolerant, and capricious, and it hurt her to see that, perhaps, he felt like he didn't exist.

Because he was good, he was a hard worker, and he only had eyes for her. It had always been like that with him. During their courtship, and even after they had gotten married, the way he used to look at her was special.

Now, he had become a bit whiny, kept more to himself... didn't share anything. He didn't talk about his friends, or about work... But why should she suspect anything?

She had to believe him. She too was responsible for this situation. She was a woman full of imagination, but in this case, where did it get her? Rather than helping her to escape from the tedium and from things she really didn't like, this special facet of hers was pushing away the man of her life. Her great love, her only love. And so, she returned to the marital bed, and she sang once more when she got up in the morning.

She thought herself happy. She wished more than anything to be happy, so she ignored her husband's tardiness and the scent that she did not recognize and which she was unable to name. She didn't like it, but she would remain coherent and avoid thinking about anything that would not make her happy.

So she received Arturo, with her long hair well-brushed, her lips painted red, and with a touch of makeup; the way he used to like, once upon a time.

She invented a story, told by the fairies that saw fit to lend her pretty novels.

She wiggled into that floral skirt which, snug at the waist, had so delighted the man of her life, in those happy times.

# XII

Ana felt she couldn't handle it all. She was overwhelmed, and it took her a while to understand why at a particular moment her mother would smother her with kisses and tell her pretty things, and later not remember what she had said, much less shower her with praise.

She had become the victim of an intense see saw which served as the foundation of everything in her life. Ana felt utterly helpless, yet she carried so many responsibilities... really, what was happening? How far could this situation go?

She used to have so many plans for the two of them. But now... now her mother... her mother was sick, suffering from Alzheimer's, a disease which sweeps everything away and kills you little by little. Wearing you down, like that drop of water which slowly, year after year, wears a hole into the stone basin of the fountain.

Ana read everything she could get her hands on, and in her free time she would sit beside her mother and tell her about what was going on in her life. Her problems. And sometimes, she would answer, completely coherent. But other times... on other occasions, she could hardly find answers, and in their place would be that empty grin which seemed to ask, "What are you telling me? What are you talking about?"

# XIII

But... some months went by... perhaps a year. And one day, when she had gotten out first from the high school, she thought of going to visit him at the office. Maybe they could dedicate a few minutes to themselves, take a walk or have a coffee. She wanted to give him a surprise, today, while their daughter was busy with her private classes.

She climbed the stairs and entered the office with the sign on the door that read: "Enter without knocking".

She entered a room which she already knew well.

Right away, a young woman came out of Arturo's office. She didn't recognize her, and that surprised her so much... so much that a cold sweat washed over her and, for a few moments, her vision became blurry. She turned pale and stuttered...

"I'm looking for Arturo."

"Oh. Is he expecting you?"

"I imagine not."

"You'll have to make an appointment. Here, I'll give you his card, if you wish to speak with him. At any rate, I can give you an appointment."

"I'm... I'm his wife."

Laura could see the young woman's eyes widen, her gaze resting upon her for a few moments. Those few moments, however, felt like hours to each of Laura's senses.

"Well, you see... he had to go out, but I'll tell him that you were here. My name is Mónica."

"It's a pleasure."

She didn't know how, or perhaps wasn't able, to say anything else. She turned around, opened the door which was left ajar, and retreated down the stairs.

She went out onto the street. She didn't know where she was. She didn't recognize this street where, when they were first married, she had waited so many times for her beloved Arturo. She didn't recognize it because her vision was so blurry it made her stagger. She was aware of the chattering of her teeth, which wouldn't stop.

She didn't care that passersby in the street were staring, nor did she know how to get home.

What had happened for her husband not to tell her he had a new person in the office? Why hadn't he told her to come by and pick him up in such a long time?

She couldn't see where she was going because the tears welled up and kept her from discerning the route back home. She opened the door to her house, but had no idea of how she had arrived there.

She left the keys on the dresser and made it to the bathroom. She began to vomit, and to cry, and to howl until her voice was hoarse, until she thought that some intruder must have followed in behind her, because her ears no longer recognized her own voice.

She went out of her mind for a moment, and like a wounded animal, looking for a way out of its own cage, she paced the house, back and forth, a prisoner of her anxiety.

Finally, she sat down on the sofa. A few hours had passed since she climbed those stairs in order to give her husband a surprise ...

The doorbell rang, and just as she was about to open, she realized she had not picked up her daughter, who must have finished her classes some time ago.

She opened the door with her face a mess, leaving the friend who had brought her daughter home by the hand speechless.

"Ana, honey... what's happened? You didn't answer the phone, you didn't come to pick up the girl, like you always do, and... for God's sake! What's wrong?"

"No... it's nothing. I just don't feel very well, and I dozed off. Must have been the heavy lunch ... Oh! I am so sorry... I'm sorry... I'm sorry..."

"Don't worry; the important thing is that you get better. It was no problem whatsoever for me to fetch Ana, you know that. We live next door to each other, and I always go to pick up my boy. Don't worry about me. But you... you are making me a bit nervous. You've been crying, and you look really, really bad. Should I call someone? The doctor? Arturo...? Have you called Arturo?"

"No. Don't worry. I'm fine, and he, he... he'll be home soon."

"Let me know if you need me, okay?"

And then, Laura hugged the little girl and told her over and over how sorry she was.

"It won't ever happen again, baby."

"It's okay, Mommy. It's okay."

Time moved forward, very slowly. She demanded a reasonable explanation, otherwise... otherwise... "But, what can I do?" she thought. "God help me, I feel so alone. The only thing keeping me together has broken."

A key turned in the door and then, Laura sat down on the sofa and quickly scooped up a newspaper which had been lying on the table for a few days.

"Hi, honey..."

She hadn't expected those words. To tell the truth, she hadn't expected to hear any words. Or maybe she did... or... And then she broke down and began sobbing uncontrollably.

He took her by the waist and hugged her, and in what appeared to be a quite affectionate and loving tone, he said:

"Shhhhhh... What's the matter? Tell me... what happened?"

She felt the tenderness, he was so sweet. She was not aware of how it happened, but she opened up her heart and asked him why he had changed secretaries and hadn't said anything to her. She asked him a thousand questions, her face twisted up, and her mouth made grotesque shapes, now like this... now... like that. She was all tears, and in her heart she was hoping for a convincing explanation.

She was praying he would convince her, so she would not have to see what awaited her in the event of an extreme situation.

"I just had to visit a client, and I thought I wouldn't get back to the office. I want... I would like it if we went out for dinner tonight. I think we need a night out, together."

"Oh, really? That's what you want? Today, of all days? Today? And where is Miss Lupe? What, she's no longer there to receive your clients? Why have you changed secretaries without telling me about it? I made the biggest fool of myself! You could at least have informed me..."

"I don't see why I have to tell you everything I do at work. I don't understand. I suppose you have to keep me informed about all the changes they make at the high school? Well? Tell me... Something as unimportant as this... you're making way too big a deal out of it.

I replaced Miss Lupe, because she was getting up in years. Or hadn't you noticed that she would soon be up for retirement? She retired. That's all it was, and of course... I had to find someone to replace her. No? Or, do you also want to give your personal stamp of approval for each person who works with me?

The truth is you are unbearable. You've got birds in your head. Your mother said you have always been very imaginative. You have always daydreamed, and as you have said yourself, without the magic of imagination there is no life. So what good does imagining do if it causes you pain? I am sure you think between that woman, that... Mónica and me there is something going on. Give me a break..."

Six months after that fateful day when she discovered the changes in the office, Laura's marriage ended. In the end, after many tries, she knew with absolute certainty that the great love of her life had become too attached to his Mónica. And when she put his bags out, in the Seventies, in that difficult decade when divorce had not yet arrived to this country, a separation marked a person for life.

Now she only had Ana, and Ana would be her support and her whole life.

# XIV

**Death is something we should not fear, because,
while we are, death is not, and when death is, we are
no longer.**

**Antonio Machado**

It was a rainy day, and the rain left streaks on the window. Laura's eyes opened again and again.

The wrinkled brow made her look older than she really was. Her eyes were half-shut.

She was dainty. Like every morning, she sat by the large window and admired the natural beauty of the park. It reminded her of the scents of her childhood, that wonderful childhood which she had loved so much and which today... she still loved?

She was still pretty. Her features were sweet, like herself. Even her gestures were distinguished, like in the way she would wipe away those tears which for some reason, slipped down her face.

Her favorite dresses were the ones with the flower prints. Her caretaker thought that it must have something to do with her rural origins, although, if she had really stopped to think about it, the prints really should have been of birds.

Yes. Birds. As Laura herself had told her when she was still completely coherent, that word was what her parents and friends had so often repeated around her since her childhood days, because her dreaming spilled over the banks of any kind of consistent reality.

Laura's disease had gotten worse, and she had arrived at the phase in which she had no elasticity. The rigidity of her muscles prevented her even from walking. That is why, every morning, Ana and Helena would sit her in the wheelchair.

Her friends did not come to see her very often unless they were invited to do so, because they felt like intruders in a home where that friend who left them was no longer.

One day, at Ana's request, Arturo had come to visit. She had known her father wished for that contact with all his heart. He entered the room, downcast, and it even looked as if he had cried.

Laura's eyes opened wide and she began to moan, turning away from him. Then, complete silence:

"Laura... I... you don't know how sorry I am this has happened to you. I want, I would like to tell you that... that I would have liked to have been by your side, taking care of you, and, of course... to have shared our daughter, Ana.

I was so young. We were so young, and many times, life takes us down paths which in the end, don't take us anywhere," he told her while taking her hands in his; Laura seemed to be looking out into infinity.

"I wish so much that you would say something... During those first years of our... living apart, we shared conversations about our daughter. After her communion... since her communion, we haven't seen each other, not even...

I can't tell you that I am sorry about everything that has happened. I have, well, you know, two other children, and I am still married... but... but I am so sorry that it couldn't have been us, you and I, who stayed together for all their lives ...

Laura, sweetheart... Look at me, and tell me you forgive me. Tell me something..."

She looked like a woman made of wax, her face staring straight ahead, and her eyes fixed on one thing, then another... until they finally fell upon Arturo, her gaze intense, and reflecting both bereavement and mistrust.

There was no trace of that love she had felt years ago. There was nothing but a tangle in her head and a stabbing pain in her heart.

"Dad... Don't talk any longer. Don't cry. I already told you it would be a bitter pill for all of us, when we agreed on the visit. I imagined you wouldn't be able to converse at all; because, at times, it seems she is completely aware, she evens follows the dialogues, but other times ... other times... you have what's happening today. She leaves. She's absent.

"Mom... Mama... my father has come to see you... Do you know who he is?"

"Yes. He's... he's a... a bastard," she said, and she struggled to get up out of the chair. Having gotten to her feet, she proved to be surprisingly strong, rejecting any help and pushing Ana aside with one arm. She then attempted to leave, running down the hall, until her brief flight ended with a fall which didn't appear to give her cause to complain.

That had happened some time ago, but now, and with each passing day, everything was becoming more complicated.

She was no longer... her. She had changed even more, and it seemed as though an impostor had taken over her body. When she no longer took an interest in her personal hygiene, Helena and Ana, realized just how fast the Alzheimer's had progressed. She didn't care whether she wore a floral dress or nothing at all.

She no longer walked. These days, Ana and Helena would lift her up and carry her around, though sometimes they required a nurse to come and lend a hand.

In spite of her mood swings, she continued to smile. All her life she had smiled.

"Why do you always lavish smiles on us?" she would hear all her life.

"Really, it comes from the heart, but maybe it has to do with the fact that I like to feel accepted, like when I was a little girl and I left the country schoolhouse to go to school in the city ... I felt so lost...," she would answer. That is, when she didn't just offer up another smile.

That day when she truly opened her heart, shortly after that conversation with the doctor, when she didn't have the courage to hear what awaited her, her world caved in around her.

But from that very moment on, she lived with the understanding that there would be no escape for her, that she was destined to endure the most difficult challenge of her life. She was condemned to escape from her body and allow today's memories to be taken by the silence and the rubber erasers.

That sensation flooded her soul.

Time went by, some months, perhaps a year...

There had been a certain stuttering, words that seemed to have abandoned her dictionary, obsessions... yes.

She had again visited the Doctor... her sentence was confirmed. Some prescriptions and a drug to slow down the inevitable had brought about some improvement.

She still felt young, and she decided that she was not going to wait about and be an easy prey. She decided she had a present and that she could not spend the little time she had left waiting to have her head lopped off by incoherence. But, what could she do? Dream. Yes. She would live out a dream, far from this place, and then she made her daughter a party to her plan.

She had talked it over with Ana, who, curious and not wishing to contradict her, applauded her decision. Both knew that fictions and realities can give shape to an entire life, and in her case... maybe it would be the best thing for both. For her to be enthusiastic and working to keep her hopes up was the way.

"Mom... you really haven't lived. I think it's the best thing you can do. By the way, are you taking me along? Would you like me to accompany you?"

"No, baby. I don't need you. I think it's good for me to go alone for fifteen days or so. In fact, I'm leaving my job. I'm going to ask for a leave of absence, but I won't tell them why. I don't want my students, or the professors themselves, to get the wrong idea about me. A lot of times, if you think someone is not well, they look bad to you even when they are well, you understand what I mean?"

"Perfectly, Mom. You do what you think is best. For me, whatever you do will be the right thing. You know that..."

She requested a leave of absence ...

"Mr. Roza. Don't misunderstand me if I wish to leave the high school. It's not that I am not happy here. But I have a personal problem, and I need to take some time off, or leave my position open forever. I don't mind."

"Laura... you can't leave us now, in the middle of the year. Can't you see it's a huge inconvenience for us?"

"I know. But it is something I must do. Don't ask me anything else. Please. I will sign all the letters of resignation that are necessary. Even if it means leaving my job indefinitely. I repeat..., don't ask me anything else."

"Have you thought this over carefully? You've been with us for so many years. The Philosophy course... there is no one like you. The students are happy with you, and even you yourself have said, time and again, that these classes are a comfort to you."

"Yes. I know."

"Are you sure you'll be able to get by without working? I just don't want you act impulsively, without thinking it over carefully."

"I have sufficient resources with which to live out the rest of my life; which, by the way, may not be very long. It might get quite complicated, you know? That is why I would like you to sign my leave, or my dismissal, or my voluntary layoff... whatever you wish. It is all the same to me, really."

And that is how Laura extricated herself from her classes and started a new life, though this worried her daughter, who couldn't help feeling some misgivings about her decision.

"I told you that you hadn't lived, but that doesn't mean you have to leap headfirst into life. For God's sake. Are you in that much of a hurry?"

"Yes. Dreaming is easy, sweetheart. I have always had more than enough imagination."

She woke up early and decided to not think of anything negative, at least for a while. She would try hard to forget that sentence handed down to her some time ago. It was quite possible that they were mistaken, or, even if that were not the case, perhaps the Fates would grant her the chance to avoid suffering from anything, and she would live to see the grandchildren she so hoped for. She could begin gathering stories which would make waiting for the bitter end more agreeable.

She put on a green skirt and a blouse with green and white stripes. The black shoes perfectly matched the bag on which she had just spent a good part of her Christmas bonus. On top of that, she wore a wool coat the same color as the bag and the shoes.

She had put on makeup – perhaps a bit more than usual – and, when it was how she liked wanted, she went down to the street.

It was quite cold out, and the idea of heading for where the weather was nice left her with a smile on her face.

She imagined a parenthesis in her life. She wished to forget her entire past, including... including the fact that she had a daughter – she wanted to be free, and she leapt at the chance to have this adventure, to travel alone. What else are dreams for?

She had a right to take some time to feel all the suffering she had been through ... because isn't it suffering, knowing that life's doors have shut before you when you are only twenty-seven years old and your husband leaves you for the first woman who makes herself available? Isn't it suffering to have to go along a path without being able to look around you, to be driven by something like the blinders her horse had, when she was a little girl?

Because, in those years, society did not look kindly upon that which was not considered correct. That was why she hadn't desired to have another man come into her house; she hadn't wanted her daughter to have a father who wasn't her real father...

And now, right now, she realized time lost can never be recovered. And what could she do? "I will fly. That's it, I will fly!"

She was free, and the ideas which would allow her to trace out a story were still available to her. It would be a story, a history that she had never lived, one which she had a right to live, even if... even if she never left the living room of her home next to the park.

And then, she held on tightly to that bit of magic hidden in her soul, and she took off flying.

At Ranón Airport the hustle and bustle was constant. The suitcases in front and behind never stopped, and there were children, elderly and middle-aged people waiting in line to board.

Laura's friends came with her to see her off. No one had known of her plan until a few days before. When she told them, they made it clear that they did not think her flying alone was a good idea. She thought it would be nice to play Russian roulette, to take a chance on a new project, before everything ended for her.

There were no delays in boarding, and, after the kisses goodbye, Laura settled into her seat.

She had asked for a window seat, and, once she made herself comfortable in her seat, she felt regret at having travelled so little. She had never had the opportunity, because life had not been very generous with her; but then, she thought, what if it had, and she had wasted those opportunities?

She took out a book and began to read. She had a bookmark with her which prominently featured a picture of the Cathedral of Oviedo. She cracked a smile. She thought of how many times she had entered the Cathedral to ask Saint Salvador to help her pass her classes, when she was a student in the city.

She started to read. The book was fairly long, some 300 pages, and it was not easy to read. The print was small, and, above all, the plot was fraught with complexities. She dozed off, the book slipping out of her hands. So, in the end, time passed in the blink of an eye, and she arrived in Tenerife Sur in what seemed to be only a few seconds.

She looked again in her bag to be sure she had brought the medicine they had prescribed for her, for possible dizzy spells and forgetfulness.

She saw the tube of pills, and she gave it a wink. Getting them to prescribe the pills had not been easy – she had had to have a long conversation with those doctors who would neither confirm nor deny her fate. But now, in her hands she had – the remedy? – and she didn't want to dwell on the negative, much less feel sorry for herself.

Two and a half hours, and the plane had already touched down.

As the plane came in for a landing, Laura contemplated the buildings and the edges of the Island itself. She felt good. She felt free and convinced that what she was doing was right. And a smile beamed on her face.

The wait for her bags took a long time. And it took so long because it had not arrived at the correct baggage carousel. She registered a complaint at the appropriate counter, and, leaving without her bag, she left for the Hotel.

She took a taxi. She had not previously arranged transportation, since she wanted to live a full experience right from the start. Taking a risk. But then, wasn't living itself a risk?

"I would like to go, please, to... wait a moment while I look at the card... one moment... yes, to the Costa Adeje Grand Hotel."

"Right away. It won't take us long. Would you like me to turn on the air conditioning?"

"If you like. At any rate, it's fine like this. Thank you."

"You have chosen a nice hotel. It is supposed to be quite comfortable, it's very nice."

"Oh! it was the travel agency that organized everything for me. I had no idea. I am not used to travelling."

"I hope you have a nice time."

"Thank you very much. I'll do my best."

The truth is that when she saw the hotel, she was impressed. Regal staircases and countless rooms, halls, swimming pools, gardens, palm trees... everything wonderfully exquisite.

At the reception desk, she explained the problem she had had with her luggage. She was told that, nearby, there was a shopping center, in case she needed anything urgently, and they informed her when things like this occurred, it did not take long for them to bring the luggage.

And so it was, and in no time at all she had settled into that marvelous place, the temperature at a comfortable eighty degrees, neither stifling nor cool.

She took a shower while talking with Ana and let her know she was already living a life of "pure luxury".

"Mom... keep your phone with you at all times, because I want to talk with you, okay? You know how many times we have talked about this. Al-ways-han-dy."

"I will, baby girl."

She put on her blue dress, made from the Chinese silk an acquaintance had brought back from a trip there. A posh seamstress, as they used to refer to her, had made it for her, but the truth is she had never put it on before now.

The sandals were not very pretty, but they did not clash with the dress in the least. The pearl necklace and earrings were set off nicely by a gold bracelet she had almost never worn.

The bracelet had belonged to her mother and it was given to her when she turned eighteen. The memory made her feel good, and, suddenly, she thought that perhaps her parents' essence, a part of them she would recognize, a part which had never died, was there with her in that heavenly hotel in Tenerife.

She went down to the lounge and ordered a mojito. She remembered having had one once, and now she wanted to know how that memory smelled. They served it to her with a lot of ice and mint, which is why the color green stood out from among the rest of the colors, and then she smelled the green and knew that her father would be by her side even if she could not see him. And she knew that her dress was blue and smelled like home. And she felt protected by her parents.

Yes. Her parents were there with her, in the midst of her dreams. After all, don't they say that those with the disease tend to remember the distant past more intensely than the relative present? This was the moment to think of them and to live out a story that was built to order.

No. Contrary to the concept most people have of the over-protected, spoiled only child, Laura had always shown character; as a girl, as a young woman and as an adult. She was not weak or needy. Not in the least. She was just... sensitive, straightforward... and perhaps a bit committed to folks in need. Although, now that she thought about it... it had been quite some time since she had dedicated herself to helping others.

And she found herself lost in thought, with Dad and Mom and the very green mojito, when he arrived:

He was a big, tall, strong fellow with graying hair. He approached her and said something which she could not make out.

"Excuse me? I don't understand what you said..."

"Oh! *Sorry*[3]. It's just that I thought you didn't speak Spanish and so I spoke in English. I am sorry... You see, you are so blonde, and I thought you must be American... My name is Tommy Rich, and I am from Nottingham."

"Well, as you can see, hair dye works miracles... My name is Laura, and I am Spanish. From Gijón."

"Yiyón... oh, where is that?"

"In Asturias. In the North of Spain."

"Nice place."

"Do you know it?"

"No, but since you are from there, I am sure *it is a very nice city*[4], because the flowers come from the plant. An ugly plant usually does not give pretty flowers."

– And then I realized I was no longer thinking, and my eyes were just popping out of my head. I was flirting with a total stranger! Because this is flirting, right? –

"Well, so... here I am, having a soft drink."

– I made a point of telling him. –

"If you were to see me drinking alcohol, you would surely think I was easy prey and... Whew, I feel quite warm. Who would have thought...!"

"A soft drink? What kind?"

---

3 NT: In English in the original text.

4 Idem

"Pineapple."

"Oh! What a good idea. Miss! A pineapple[5] drink, please!"

Almost immediately, a glass arrived, its contents an off yellow color. They looked at each other and fell silent.

She got rid of him as soon as she could, and, of course, she did not have dinner in the dining room that night. She went up to her room, and they brought her a sandwich, a coca-cola and a tomato salad, and she ate in front of the television. She ate everything except the tomatoes... she did not care too much for tomatoes, and she rethought back to the ones her father used to pick. Those were big, and not very smooth. She remembered how strange she had thought it when he would often pick them from the climbing vine when they were still green.

"Sweetheart... I do that because if they stay on the vine too long, they run the risk of being spoiled by a disease that leaves them with blotches."

And when she heard that, she thought it would be a good idea if they all rotted. She had never liked them. That is why those cherrys now lay alone in the middle of the tray, so small they reminded her of bonsai tomatoes.

It always hurt her to see a bush that should be large and leafy reduced to a replica and far removed from its origins.

The next day nothing happened beyond her walks and her amazement at feeling so good with herself, so far from home.

And the following day proved to be a carbon copy of the day before.

She sunbathed covered with sun protection. She spread the contents of the tube slowly and thoroughly, over every part of her skin exposed to the air.

She took long walks along the Costa Adeje; she hiked up the hill, alongside the Castle on the sea, so she could have a bird's-eye view

5 Idem.

of the sandy beach; she breathed everything in deeply and forgot about the sentence that had been passed down to her, just as she had intended.

Yes. She had thoroughly researched the island. She was still able to go on the Internet. She had just left the high school, and she was relatively well, but... there were parts of her memory that often failed her; she believed that the real problem was when she didn't know what the object she had in her hands was used for, no matter how familiar the thing was.

But today, she was still able to think, and she was going to live intensely, because, as she believes, she had earned the right. She rebelled. After all, doesn't a wild animal fight to avoid the cage? Doesn't the snake bite when it is trod upon?

But no... she had no intention of sinking her teeth into some hapless prey. If anyone was the victim, it was Laura...

She would not allow life to swallow her up so easily.

Her cell phone rang again and again... the friends who were not aware of what she was facing were calling, horrified at her decision to run off. All the whispers and murmuring over the afternoon coffee must have been something. Maybe they thought she had run off with some man, to live an adventure.

This is the situation: in the room next door to hers, a middle-aged man was getting settled. He was tall, blond, with a neat and tidy look to him, and whenever they ran into each other, he gave her a charming smile. And another, and another...

"I'm Jorge, and you are...?"

"Laura."

"A beautiful name."

"Yours too."

Then Laura went into her room, with a faint smile on her lips. She felt young and pretty. She thought of the wonderfully gratifying feeling provoked by that man whom she had met two days ago and ran into every time she entered or left her room.

And finally, on the third day, they got together for dinner.

"What's brought you here? I am sorry if I seem impertinent with all these questions, but it's how I am. I handle public relations for a computer company, and so, you can see... well, you will see... it's a habit you pick up on the job. I ask questions, and often I blush at them, but... I stick to my guns..."

"I am here on vacation. I've been here five days. Yes. Five days, no more, and I have ten days left. I think I should have arranged to come for at least a month. I love everything, and I feel happy."

"Laura... where are you from?"

"I'm from Gijón, I'm divorced, I have a twenty-five year old daughter, and I'm a high school teacher."

"Ha ha ha..., I said to myself that you had the look of a clever lady. You knew I would ask you those questions, right?"

"Right."

"I'm from Madrid, and I travel out here to the Island from time to time. I still have a few more days here... yes, I still have fifteen days left."

"And are you... are you... married?"

"No. I was, but I've been divorced for ten years. I have two children."

"I... it's been... yes... I got divorced over twenty years ago. Thank God. I have never wanted anything more to do with men... I think I've come to hate them."

"So... does that mean you are a lesbian?"

"No, of course not. It's not that, either. I'm not a lesbian or anything at all. I have never needed anybody."

"Never? I mean... during all this time there hasn't been anyone in your life? And, anyway, there's nothing wrong with being a lesbian... really... I think."

"Of course there's nothing wrong with it, but it's just that I am a woman of extremely little passion. And as far as affection goes, I have got that covered thanks to my daughter and my closest friends."

"Oh! Of course, that is always an option. Of course, in my case, it is different. I am very passionate. I would love to be with you... I mean, intimately. I would love for you to be able to feel like a woman. It's possible you've never experienced those sensations, otherwise you surely could not have done without them for so long."

"I think you are moving very fast. It seems to me a lack... a lack of... respect, this conversation we are having. I... I've lost my appetite. I am going to leave. I am sorry, but I need to go up to my room."

As Laura dreamt, she heard Helena telling her it was time to eat.

She didn't have an appetite. She didn't feel well, and, besides, she had to stay here by the balcony. Behind the white lace curtain, there was a chair from which she had always admired the vegetation sketched out behind the glass.

There, after dinner, she used to sit and read well into the night. Her sleeplessness was an accomplice that made it possible for her to read one book after the other, day after day.

Now she was dreaming, and between dreams, she felt that stroke of pain which pierced her stomach and that trace of fear which she surely would conquer; while it was still possible...

"It is hard to recognize yourself and not admit you have recognized yourself..."

"But, really... who do you take me for?"

"Honey, I thought you were more modern. I didn't mean to offend you. But, it's just that I find it so strange that there hasn't been anyone in more than twenty years."

"You didn't offend me, you just frightened me. That is how it's been...there hasn't been anyone, and I think there never will. So you see. Those are the kind of decisions one makes in life."

"Decisions one makes in life, you say... What do you know! I mean, you hadn't met me, until today."

"Hmmm... maybe that's it."

They were having an exquisite meal, but Laura no longer had an appetite. But she felt good next to Jorge. He smelled green. Yes. Yes, of course, and that was a point in his favor. And at that moment she got up and said good night to him, then hurried off.

Half-smiling, he followed her, catching up to her at the elevator. He took her by the arm, the door opens, the two entered the elevator, and he kissed her so passionately that... that she felt something she had never felt before.

Laura, let herself go. Jorge's tongue was pressed deep inside her mouth, the door to the room opened – how, she didn't know – and the two of them were on the bed, undressing, with the blue dress flying off along with the rest of her clothing ... until all that she had left on was her mother's gold bracelet. Nothing else.

The light turned on. Jorge said:

"I want to see those green eyes of yours. I want to admire you while we make love. You're beautiful."

"I don't know what to say..." she gasped. "I don't even know how I got here... Oh, my God!"

"What's the matter?"

"Do you think that maybe... I mean... after so long... maybe it's closed up... you know..."

"Do you mean to say your hymen?"

"More or less... I mean, it's been more than twenty years, and that's a long time, don't you think? Oh! Wait..."

"Now what's the matter?"

"I forgot, my parents are here... here. What will they think when they see me like this?"

"You've got to be...!! Are your father and mother here? Here?

"I was having a mojito, and I could feel them around me..."

"Whew, what a scare you gave me, honey. You know, those mojitos work miracles... I could see you were special."

Laura blushed when she thought of her parents being able to peek into this secret story she was living, and then, she went back to looking out the window, observing how life could unfold pleasantly even when one was aware of the sentence they were facing.

And then, without any reservations, without paying any mind to the presences she had perceived, they made love.

No. There was no blood on the sheets like the first time. But there were passionate kisses, rhythmic penetrations, hands entwined and tickles of desire.

They kissed again and again, and suddenly they leaned their faces back, simply to contemplate one another. To see each other and to lose themselves in each other's eyes.

The heavens were aglow with the colored lights of desires fulfilled. There was the scent of mint and the smell of yearning.

Skin... that silken skin brushing softly against his. Their skins, perhaps, had been unconsciously looking for one another their whole lives.

Their feet intertwined, and, finally, when calm fell once more, it fell so strongly that it left them with a feeling that time had stopped.

And like this, hugged tightly, in the strong arms of this man whom she had only just met, she was overcome by sleep...

They no longer used two rooms.

The day after their first time together, they again experienced those moments of glory and ecstasy, and they sought each other again and again. And the next day...

No. That was not runaway passion between two strangers. That was love, and the feeling of love. That was the purest feeling that could invade souls so alike.

In the morning, in the shower together, they would rub up against one another, following the trails left by the shampoo bubbles.

The water followed the course of the rhythm of their desire, and after, they followed the trails left by the drops that danced about them ... One day like this, another day playing at love, becoming one, enveloped by the scent of Aloe Vera.

Jorge would take her in his arms in one, long... never-ending embrace.

They usually had breakfast together at one table which was slightly farther away from the rest of the people. They way they looked at each other, it was as if they knew everything about each other just by gazing into each other's eyes, and they smiled as if they were party to the same secret, while they held hands, their fingers mingling playfully.

The walks along the beach were accompanied by seagulls who seemed to caw love songs to them. There were small boats dotting the horizon and jostled by the waves, now saying yes, now no.

"Now yes, now no..."

"What did you say?"

"I was saying that... now you see them, now you don't... the boats, I mean. Can't you see how they are being jostled about?"

"Yes, Laura. I see them. Like life itself. We are the boats, and life jostles us about from one end to the other ... don't you think?"

"Yes. Maybe yes."

The days were marvelous, the meals were a feast for the eyes and the palate, the afternoons in the sun were a delight, and the nights, the mornings... a discovery of what it is to live. Of what it is to love. No... Love with a capital L, life's gift to them, perhaps to balance the scale of experiences.

"We'll continue to see each other, my darling... I'll go to Asturias, and we'll continue our relationship. My love, you are the best thing that has ever happened to me."

"No, Jorge. What we have must end on this island. The moment we part, it will be forever.

"I will live with the memory of this story, for all the rest of my life. But it is not possible for us to continue seeing each other. That life together that you have asked me to share will not be possible, because sometimes in life, we don't have control of the direction it takes. What we have lived together has been the greatest gift I have ever received, but, for me, what we have shared can only be a break between my past and the future that awaits me..."

"I don't understand you, Laura. I can't understand you. Do you have someone waiting for you back home? Have you been lying to me, and you have someone else? Laura... I don't think you are capable of something like that."

"Don't ask me questions that I can't answer. Darling, situations are what they are, and, today, right now, I am leaving forever."

There was a beginning and an end, which started and finished during the remaining days of that trip to Tenerife.

They day they said goodbye that morning it was gray.

They got together for breakfast. They hardly talked, and they touched each other's hands, again and again. Their fingers were intertwined, and they stared long and hard into each other's eyes. A thousand and one my loves and my darlings were heard all those days they had spent together, and now, during their farewell, it would be no different.

There was a glow in their hearts, and hearts with that glow have a battery which causes the earth to stop spinning during those romantic encounters.

They said their goodbyes at the airport. Their lives took different paths.

He desired to continue this romance; he called it unique and powerful, and he proclaimed there had never been other like it. She knew she had little time left, and the moments she had lived at his side would be enough to go on during the remaining months or years that life might grant her.

And so, during their farewell:

"Jorge... Now remember... don't come looking for me. I should not see you again."

And having said that, she hurried through passport control at the Tenerife South Airport.

She cried inconsolably and ran to the boarding gate. The hem of her red dress danced from one side to the other, as if the swaying of her body sought to sing a danceable melody.

She was anxious to board the plane, thinking that there, only there, she would find the safety and the peace she needed to come to terms with this goodbye.

"Welcome aboard, Madame... can we help you with anything?" she heard the flight attendant say at the foot of the plane, and, with that, she realized she was hiccupping as the tears streamed down her face. She simply shook her head no...

She sat on the right side of the plane. Once again, she had a window seat. She fastened her safety belt and placed her handbag on her lap for a few moments, until the flight attendant indicated that she would not be able to keep it there during takeoff. She hadn't remembered that, and she apologized, placed the bag on the floor.

She cast her gaze off into the distance and looked at that strip of land where she had known passion, where she had found the man of her dreams, when she no longer had time... to dream.

With tears in her eyes she blew a kiss, leaving two fingers pressed upon her lips, for how long she could not tell.

She dozed during the entire flight. Her eyes fluttered open a few times, only to close again, in search of that peace she so needed...

And Laura got up, opened the door and went down the stairs, her head held high, a faint smile on her lips and slippers on her feet.

Suddenly, a shudder raced up her spine and invaded the back of her head. She had confused reality with the fiction of her make-believe story, and she melted into a bitter cry and rushed up the stairs.

# XV

The days went by and Laura's life became more entangled. The continual expressions of indifference towards everything, along with the extreme emotional lows and highs. Cry, laugh. Love, perhaps hate... But what is hate? Had she ever felt hate before? Would this new circumstance induce her to feel that base, painful emotion?

Uncertainty; her now was not today. Tomorrow hardly existed, because her mind would run from projects and cling onto yesterday, and her dreams were stunted.

She would repeatedly discover proof that everything was becoming more and more complicated. From the moment the doctor asked her if she really wanted to know whether she was suffering from Alzheimers, and she answered no, she had known that the sword of Damocles was poised above her head. There would be no escape.

And one day, when she discovered that she didn't remember what a fork was called, when it was evident that she couldn't remember the name for this common, everyday object she had held in her hands all her life... she started shaking.

Thunder would rumble in the sky, and her empty gaze would reveal nothing. Or, she would appear to be absent, though, perhaps, all the thoughts that would not come out in words were bubbling deep within her.

Who can truly know the secrets of the mind, when it appears that the mind is no longer? Who probes memory, when science says memory is lost, and that which was can never be remembered coherently?

However, Laura, was prepared. She had been made aware of her horrific situation many times, and, one day, she spoke openly, with her daughter, about what was happening to her:

"Listen...I cannot ignore what is real. I can't continue hiding my situation, as if nothing were wrong, thinking that, maybe, if I don't involve you, that nothing will happen. That's why, sweetheart, I must talk to you clearly:

For some months now, very strange things have been happening to me. The little slips I didn't pay attention to, because I have always been a bit absentminded, but... I've had this smell of sorrow for some time. You know that smell of sorrow comes from the stomach. I feel like instead of a stomach, someone threw a rock in a lake, and the shock wave is expanding. In this case, the lake is here," and she indicates her waist, "and the shock wave is none other than that feeling of sorrow... of sadness which is now flooding my heart.

They've told me that in the initial phase of the disease, the patient presents symptoms of depression; although, of course, I know depressions do not necessarily have their origins in Alzheimer's. I know that all too well, but more than that, quite often, I can't find the words to speak. It's as if the whole alphabet were playing hide and seek with me.

I've also lost some capacity to feel happiness, and I become obsessed with the most unimportant things, things I am worrying about one day after another, about these ideas that just stick to my worn out neurons.

Yes, baby. I have Alzheimer's, and we have to be strong. We have to be very strong.

They say when the disease occurs in a young person – I know, I am not young, but I'm not so old that I'm going to simply resign myself to being a prisoner and submit meekly to my fate – I mean, I'm not young, but I am too young to give up without a fight.

That is why I want to make everything I can as clear as possible, so that it is as painless as possible for everyone.

You are here, my Ana, my daughter. And in you, with you, is the person who will have to be a witness to my decline, and I only ask for understanding, for my absences and my lethargies, and, why not, for the rage they say takes over people who, like me, suffer from this disease.

I ask you to conserve the memory of my love for you. I want you to know that, even though I may appear to become and act like a stranger, I will always be Mommy, your Mommy who adores you more than anything. And for you I would not only give my one life... but a thousand lives... a million lives.

I want you to know that that I believe each of us follows his own path of evolution, and nothing happens just by chance. We all form part of a pre-established script, and certain decisions we make may result in changes to it. But, while we may jump paths, in the end one path after the other will lead us back down the road we abandoned and someday must take up again.

Ana, daughter... you and I have many things in common. We have always been so close that, one more time – and this will be the last, but not easy – I am going to ask you to do something for me:

Do you remember how many times we played at guessing each other's thoughts just by looking into each other's eyes? We have never needed words to understand one another, sweetheart, and that is why you are more qualified than anyone to be my eyes, my feet, when I... when I can't move them anymore, and my hands and, of course... my thoughts which I will no longer be able to express.

Sweetheart, you have told me many times that you felt certain that the people with this disease... that their feelings don't die. That they maintain the capacity to love, that they know and recognize much more than they are able to express.

Maybe that's why you are here, maybe fate itself has made you the way you are, and that is why you can demonstrate all that you know about the mysteries of the mind. The inscrutable mind, as you have called it so many times... But from what I can see, you have managed to see beyond what the books say, and I have great faith in your intuition and inner knowledge.

No. I don't want to tether you to my circumstances, but I do want to continue to feel, to think, to live through you, my dearest. You will have some hard work, but I won't let you down."

"Mom, for God's sake... come on, your speech is totally coherent. I haven't noticed anything strange in you... You are exaggerating things... we all have memory lapses, and stomach pain and..."

"No. The sentence has been handed down: Alzheimer's.

Some days ago, I consulted another neurologist, and he asked me a series of questions, I had to draw some hieroglyphics, he checked my reflexes, he took a look at the back of my eyes... there's no doubt. He ran a number of different tests on me...

He thought it was strange that I went by myself to see him, but he understood when I told him I only wanted to confirm what I already knew.

All of those tests, we will have to do them again, together, you and I. And the moment will come when I won't be aware, when it will seem like I don't love you, but you... you will know that is not true."

There were hugs and kisses and many tears, but after a little while they were sitting at the table, and she helped herself to the food and talked about this and that as if the conversation they had just had a few minutes ago had never happened.

Ana, stared at her plate and casually spun it around, and this did not escape Laura's attention. Suddenly, Laura felt a sharp pain, the smell of dark gray creeping over her heart which, and an immense wave of sadness swept through her soul.

She had placed all this responsibility on her poor daughter, but it didn't seem to be the best moment to relieve her of the burden she had placed upon her. It seemed so selfish on her part to do this to the girl. Girl? No. Her daughter was, of course, was no longer a child; she had covered a lot of ground in her life and still had a lot of ground ahead of her. But for Laura, her daughter would always be a part of herself.

Yes. She would have to tell Ana not to worry, that she would have someone to take care of her on a daily basis. But when Laura no longer had much time left, Ana would be her interpreter. She would wait for another day to tell her, when they were alone.

Laura's house was big. Almost as big as that great house her father had had built for them when she was only eight years old.

When she and Arturo got married, they lived for a while in a one-bedroom apartment. Later, because they both worked, they moved to a large flat in front of a park. She still lived there today.

Those houses didn't have stone steps climbing the hill, like those steps by the home where she and her parents had gone to live so many years ago.

What had always been a part of her was that beautiful grove and the multitude of flowers. Jasmine in winter, and roses, carnations, wisteria and ivy in the summer.

Laura had a special admiration for Nature. Whether it was present was not important. Her imagination would carry her as far as she had to go. She liked the smells... the smells of a spring evening, of the delicate heat of summer, of snow, of fallen leaves... those nights when she would sneak out to the meadow, lying in the grass without caring if it was damp and gazing at the stars, while a feeling of freedom coursed through her body.

In the distance, she could hear the bells around the necks of the cows she was imagining, and that helped bring her back to her unique childhood, when she just a little girl and had not yet started going to school in the city. She contemplated herself, that round-faced girl who would often stop in front of that anthill, contemplating the intense, endless work of its residents, who carried loads upon their backs which seemed to be four times their size.

She loved the feel of the storm and the rain through the windowpanes. That heavy rain striking the glass would produce tones which rang out like notes from a piano. And later, the sun.

She remembered herself living experiences which only existed in her memory and dreaming that someday she would be important. At what, she didn't know, but she felt she would be important in the future. And so it was... she would often laugh when she remembered those wings of hers poised for flight. She had been important in her house, or at least so she thought... and she arrived at the silly notion that it is better to conform and avoid suffering.

But today, today I am prepared. I am going to fight to have my feelings understood, because Ana, my baby, is going to know intuitively what I am feeling but cannot say. Because you, you may erase my memories, but they are recorded in the precious box of experiences, so that no one can ever erase what has been written by me. Because my daughter is going to know that I will never stop loving her, much less stop smiling. I swear it. Because every one of my feelings exists outside of my mind and shall be immutable.

Now we are face to face. I have been waiting for this moment for some time.

# XVI

Philosophy is the cultivation of the mental faculties.
It uproots our vices and prepares the spirit to receive
the appropriate seed.

**Epicurus**

The candles were crowded together, one behind the other, on the round cake. The table was set, elegantly complemented by the Bohemian crystal wine glasses which reigned over the rest of the glassware. Fifty-five candles. The cake seemed to show off its roundness. It was a tarta Gijonesa, tasting of turrón and burnt sugar. It was her special dessert, and for that reason it was part of today's surprise. There was more... gifts which now adorned her neck and ears. She had put them on, and now they applauded the fact that she had been unable to blow out the candles, pretending it had been a performance on her part, perhaps to make her believe she was still herself.

The linen tablecloth, yellow... yellow, what does yellow smell like? And then Laura, from her branch, saw herself inhale with all her might, thinking that she had never assigned a scent to that color, and she breathed in, deeply... even more deeply, only to afterwards turn pale. Her pituitary registers the scent of defeat, the smell of life racing downhill. And then, it occurred to her that one guest had come to this, her fifty-fifth birthday, the guest who, though expected, turned out to be for her the most intriguing.

In the morning, Helena always rushed to arrive to the house. She would pant alarmingly, although they later discovered that she would start breathing heavily just as she entered the building, in an effort to excuse her tardiness.

Helena had come to Spain some years ago, from Russia, in search of some peace for her stomach, as she would often say.

Her family had remained behind in Novosibirsk, her hometown, and it was up to her to send a good part of what she earned back home to support her family:

"Life is being very difficult, Missus, and we have no way to educate my daughter Irina's boys. And my husband, the poor man, he has no work either, and you see... sixty years, and me, going around the world," she would say, or lament.

"Pardon me, Miss Ana, but I missed the bus, and well, you know... how did the Missus sleep?"

"Well. The truth is, as you can see, she almost doesn't do anything anymore. You know... talk to her, since she still may be able to understand you.

"Give her a kiss. She always receives any show of affection with a smile. If she doesn't smile with her lips, she will smile with her eyes.

"For lunch, well, you know already... purée, very light. It's getting quite difficult for her to swallow, and so... I'll have to go the pharmacy and get a syringe with a wide mouth. It's the only way to feed her.

"Yes... I know you think I repeat myself, one day after the other, but it is important, that while I am working, that you do what I would do, if it were possible for me to be with her, alright?"

"Alright, Miss. Have a very nice day."

"You too, Helena."

The days passed, one after the other. Regular walks with Laura in her wheelchair. Greetings from the neighbors and the questions they shouted at her ...

"So... How is the Missus today? You look very pretty. The truth is you look stunning!!!"

Then, Helena would remind them that Mrs. Laura, was ill, but, of course... she was not deaf, and then she thought to herself, "Why do people think, when we don't understand, that it is necessary to shout?"

Laura always wore a flower. A flower from among those she had always loved so much. During those walks, Helena or Ana, depending on the moment, would pick a small branch from the park, or a small leaf from a hedge. Until almost her final days, she would receive those small gifts with a smile. Perhaps that smile was one of gratitude meant for life itself, for having given her the chance to admire its creation, and for having been born in the country, her beloved country.

"Ana... I think you mentioned once that your mother asked you to interpret her gaze ... Pardon, but you go in such a hurry... you work so much... I understand, but... it seems to me you have forgotten to look behind her eyes. I think you have to interpret something," Helena told her.

Ana, turned pale, reproached herself a thousand, a million times. She asked herself how she could have forgotten such an important responsibility. Had the moment arrived? But why was hadn't she been aware that for some time now her mother only stammered, unable to speak at all?

"It can't be true... Mom... forgive me... Mom!! I'm sorry... I'm so sorry."

And with that she began to wail, as if her life were being ripped away from her, and she ran to hug her, to cling to her lap and listen to the beating of her heart.

"How could I have forgotten you?"

And, now, with that question still ringing in her ears, Ana penetrated her mother's eyes, and went beyond. Ana experienced uncertainty and sorrow, and she felt rather ashamed about having broken through those physical barriers in order to gain access to that hidden place her mother had said she would someday be able to enter.

And then, daughter and mother began a dialogue, without words, when they could no longer speak, as had been the case for some time.

Ana felt bad, because she had been absorbed by her work, and she almost hadn't noticed the deterioration that had ravaged this woman, her mother. It was a dialogue without words, without sounds, without the need to express anything physical:

"Oh, Mom! I thought the disease would be slower, and I didn't keep in mind what we had talked about. I'm sorry for having been so absorbed in my own life... I'm sorry, Mom."

And then her green eyes began to speak:

"Sweetheart, don't suffer. There is nothing you can do. I am fine, I am aware of what is happening to me at every moment, though my mind does not overcome all the obstacles, and doesn't know how to say this or that. I want to talk, but, in fact, the words that come out are incoherent. And, some time ago I tried reading, but I don't remember that I have to read the book in front of me: I open it and look at the letters, but a moment passes and already I am unable to recall what I have just read. My mind is useless, but something in me knows I cannot do it any better. Something in me knows, though I cannot put it into words. Sometimes, I want to tell Helena that my leg hurts, or my arm, and I know what it is that hurts me, but I can't put anything into words, because I don't know how.

I am hungry and I know I am hungry, but the words don't come out then either.

Other times you give me something to eat and I only feel like vomiting...

Baby, I want you to know that I am still here, dressed up as someone who doesn't know how say what is happening to her, and who doesn't understand anything. But I am still here, by your side, by the side of those who have already gone, and my feelings are as alive as they have ever been.

Only my neurons are going, but... who says our neurons are what steers a human being's life?"

"Mom, what can I do for you?"

"My daughter... wait. Look into my eyes when you think you can understand me. You need serenity. Me, well, as you can see... I am still here. I am not going anywhere. Maybe this life right now is upsetting to you, but I don't wish that to be so. There is nothing else I can do. At any rate, I don't have much time left.

I am sorry I have these mood swings, and I can imagine how difficult it must be for you, but I can't help it. I can't avoid getting angry, just like I can't help feeling euphoric when I don't have any reason to be. I don't know.

Most of the time I wander about. There is nothing I can hold onto, and a chasm is opening under my feet. My feet, what are they? They are part of me, but they are not me. And who am I? All I know is that I smell yellow. And that leaves me with the feeling of a horrible knot in my stomach.

Sweetheart... I just want you to understand me and to know how to look behind me, because behind me, that is where I am."

"I will look, Mom, don't worry. I will always be by your side, just like your friends who are here, like that childhood friend of yours, who came up from Valladolid last week, remember? Because you should know that, even though we practically have no family, many of our neighbors come to see you, and your friends are always around, all of us are with you. They call you on the phone, and they visit you every chance they get. But don't ever forget how much I love you..."

"No sweetheart, no. all of them have gone, leaving behind only impostors."

# XVII

If death were not the prelude to another life, our
current life would merely be a cruel joke.

Mahatma Gandhi

This time the cake was long. The mold was not round, and now
even the toast with champagne was staged. Laura's – my mother's
– friends had come to share what perhaps would be the final toast,
alerted by the sad portents that indicated the end was growing near.

I had them come because it was possible she was still aware of
everything happening around her; when I penetrated into her interior,
she would claim that it was so.

Mom was at the head of the table, sitting in her wheelchair. She
did not blink as she observed the fifty-six lit candles. With a vacant
stare and a certain amount of fear, she watched the tiny flames; it was
as though this were the first time her retinas had ever perceived them.

Her skin was white. It had been shielded from the sun to avoid
being damaged. Her gaze would sometimes vanish, and then, for days
on end, it would be impossible for me to interpret her thoughts, until,
suddenly, her gaze would return to and she would be herself again.

It is curious how life teaches us to live. It is curious how we had
gotten used to living with this sad circumstance which, until then, had
been unimaginable.

Every day there was the same ritual.

Helena would get her up from the bed and carefully place her in her chair. Her strength was no longer up to this task, so we had asked an assistant to come and help, because I have to go to work.

Some days, I would be moved to tears when I felt she was again there with me. I would sense that the stranger she had become had left, and that my mother had returned once again. Because, she would come and go.

I will always remember how often, over the course of the disease, I would say to her:

"Hello, Mom. How did you sleep?"

"What did you say? Did you call me Mom? How dare you – I never had any children in my life. Of all the nerve."

And on days like that I would cry, and that night I would cry, and the following day and the next one too. And I would look into her eyes again and again, finding no one. My mother, the essence of my mother, was not there, and then I would burst out crying, screaming, made an orphan by someone who had not died. And all the cuddling, the caresses, all the love she had given me just dissolved, like a cloud that gradually loses its shape.

I remember how coquettish she had become, how she loved to look at herself in the mirror, but how many times she failed to recognize herself, I lost count.

"Who is that? What is she doing here?"

"Mom, that's you! See how pretty you are?"

"Ma'am, that is you, you don't realize how well you young you still look, and pretty, pretty," Helena would say.

"That's me? What foolishness! I don't understand how you could have done this to me. My whole life I have been quite generous. I have been a first-class citizen, and the two of you, are mocking me... pigs, the two of you. Pigs."

Because, while my mother often could not find the right words to express herself, when the opportunity arose to swear and curse, she had a whole battery of harsh adjectives at her disposal.

I cried so much, so often, for so many years; I cried as many tears as I had cried during my entire life. It is so sad to lose someone who is alive and there beside you and yet not living. There simply are no words to define it.

Towards the end, she was no longer able to walk. She could not take even a single step, so we would put her in her wheelchair and take her out for a walk. She would look around, with a certain malice reflected in her eyes. She was afraid and she with each passing day she felt more and more threatened.

At first, when she lost control of her sphincters, she felt terrible and ashamed, but it wasn't long before she came to no longer care in the least; she was not aware of the care and dedication she was receiving from those around her, and whenever our heads were near, she would even pull on our hair.

Some days she would laugh and laugh; she would roar with laughter and nod her head for us to join in. When we did, she would look at us as if she were having visions.

And me, I kept looking into her eyes, as she had instructed.

She had prepared herself to confront the disease, and she had worked out all the details, with the aim of not losing her identity.

After the day on which I struck up that first communication, gaze to gaze, I couldn't say what had happened to me; no matter how often I tried, I couldn't find her. Until one day, when her bones had already become rigid and she had difficulty swallowing, I saw her again.

It was spring. The sky was blue, and, as she used to say, blue smells like home. Suddenly, she was there.

There it was, that gaze; it was the same old her, and our communication, which had been missing began again.

I said, "Mom," and she answered:

"Tell me, baby."

"Why have you been away for so long? I followed your instructions, and I looked into your eyes every day. You were never there, and my heart has walked alone, heavy... shattered."

"It's just that I was living my experience."

"Yes, fine... but while you were living that experience of yours, I was suffering because I thought you had left."

"Even so, it's not like that. I was behind my eyes. I was behind all this sad adversity, that part of the reality that is my lot."

"So why didn't you come? I begged you, and you didn't show up."

"Sweetheart... I have always loved you. I have always loved you all. Haven't you noticed how I planted a kiss on your face every time you asked me? Haven't you seen how I kissed everyone who has loved me and whom I still love?"

"Yes. I have seen it."

"You have to keep in mind, always, that while the apparent coherence has left, the feelings are still present. Because the mind is one aspect of life, and the soul is another. The soul possesses an entire spectrum of feelings, and these feelings never die, even after the neurons have destroyed the intellect.

You must always keep in mind, dearest Ana, that anything and everything may be altered or destroyed, but feelings never perish. Because feelings, just like colors, form a part of the magic of life. And the feeling of love, of life, of light, smells of orange.

And orange represents that sun which has shone brilliantly and now sets, though it lives on, in another place, even if you cannot see it. It represents that light which illuminates, with the oblique rays of destiny. It represents that bet on permanence.

Nothing is forever, dear Ana. Nothing is forever except for permanence, which never ends, though the body is stilled.

Don't be afraid when I go, because I will not have left entirely. Because I will continue to be by your side.

You know? I never told you this, but that time I travelled to Tenerife – seems so long ago, now – I found myself with my Dad and Mom. I saw them, I swear it."

"You saw them in Tenerife?"

"Yes, there in my hotel."

"But, are you trying to tell me that their death was nothing more than pantomime, that they moved to where the sun was in order to live a better life?" I was joking with her. "And where did you see them exactly?"

"Sweetheart, I could feel them there, with me while I was drinking a mojito."

"Mom! You are not even behind your eyes! And here I thought I was communicating with the real you ... and, instead, it's just my imagination! They should put me away."

"No, Ana. What I am telling you is much more serious than you think. In the mojito there was a great quantity of green mint. I recalled how my father smelled green to me, and how my mom smelled like laundry blue. But, now, the two of them, together, were wearing green.

No. I don't mean that they were put there in my glass like a couple of inanimate figures. No.

Simply, I recalled them, and then, they were there; I could feel their presence. I felt them beside me, and I knew, then and there, that nobody dies forever, although I had always been fairly certain that this is how it was... how it is, baby. That is how it is.

That has been one of the strongest impressions I have ever experienced in my life, and I have had many others since. Because, you know what? Behind my eyes, where the eyes rest and where life lives, that is the realm of the essences that never die. There, that is where life takes on meaning and becomes life in the fullest sense.

Never forget that the eyes see, and the Soul watches. Don't ever forget that, and don't ever be afraid of anything.

We are in the school of life. A school where we must learn from the experiences we have chosen to live out, in order later to return to our home, all the wiser.

Don't bend over backwards when someone steps on you, even though you may fall to the ground. Think always of the opportunities life has given you so that you may know how to fall. Yes, the ground is hard and cold, but the lesson you learn makes the ground cottony soft and helps you in your evolution.

I am not dead; though I appear twisted, my eyes lost in the distance, my mouth drooling, seemingly absent... don't suffer. It is not what it seems. All that you lose in your physical life, you gain in your world of energy. Because we are energy, dear daughter. And energy does not die."

"Oh, Mom! Really, I don't know if what you are saying is absurd or not. But..."

"Daughter... you smell of laundry blue, just like my mother used to smell... my mother, whom you did not get to meet. You know she passed away before you were born. And when I had you in my arms, I could see that you were the same.

I hope you never find yourself alone, sweetheart. I hope that in your next marriage you are luckier than I have been, though everything happened because it had to happen."

"Well, if you say I smell of laundry blue, so it shall be."

"So that there are never any secrets between us, I am going to tell you one I have kept to myself all this time."

"Oh? What is it?"

"On my trip to Tenerife, I met a man. His name was, and perhaps still is, Jorge."

"And?"

"Well, I felt with him what I had never felt before. I spent a few, wonderful, unforgettable days with him. I was very happy living that experience that had no future."

"Why didn't you tell me?!"

"It's good to keep some things for oneself, sweetheart."

"And you didn't stay in touch? You were still well then."

"I wasn't well, baby. Really. It lasted just as long as it had to last. I couldn't make it so that both our feelings could continue on their course, so I decided to insinuate that our romance had to stay on the island, that once I was back home, I move on again with my life."

"Mom! The way you left it, it's like someone very..."

"Listen, honey... I was not well by then, and I was well aware of it. One day at lunch I suffered an important memory lapse. No. Not a moment of absent-mindedness like the many I have had in my life. Not in the least! I had a comb in my hand, and I had no idea what it was for. That is why, that time it happened with you... that wasn't the first time I didn't know what an object was for.

Then, because I had not lost that slyness of mine – oh no! – I gracefully placed the comb in my lap, while my companion's eyes bugged out.

The same thing happened to me with the key to my room. I looked at it as if I had never before seen anything like it in all my life. What I felt was so traumatic, because that really is something important.

Those little slips, the small forgotten things, those usually happen to everyone. But what is really troublesome is when you know an object so well but you don't know what it is used for. An object with which you have always been in contact."

"And then?"

"I told him what I told him, so that he wouldn't suffer, and so that I wouldn't suffer. I had no right to set off on a love story, knowing as I did that a black destiny awaited me. A destiny as black as that hole which has carried away my history and my senses, but which never shall never be able to absorb my feelings and the lessons I have learned in life.

But, believe me. I discovered love, and that is the most beautiful thing in the world. I hope, baby, that you will be as happy as I was on that island."

# XVIII

A few days have gone by, and the wheelchair is no longer here. They have taken it away, because I no longer need it.

That day when Laura, my mother, left... I dreamed of her: She was sitting on the branch of a great tree. The tree had many branches and an intense green color. She was smiling as she swung her legs back and forth, as if she were on an imaginary swing.

In her hands, she held a small, blue box, balanced on her lap. I observed the scene from the ground, and she smiled at me, and I could hear her say to me:

You see? I have recovered my memories. They were locked away in a magic box, in which all the memories of everyone who has ever lived are kept.

Don't let it bother you, my dearest, if you think that you have let me down in some way. Don't fear – because, inevitably, my circumstances had to be lived, and you, my life, have supported me, you have done so much for me. Too much, even though to you it may seem that it wasn't enough.

Do you remember when you were a little girl, and I would tell you about the fairies? Do you remember how many times I told you that the moon was within your reach, and that you only have to believe it in order to hold it in your hands? Everything is possible, sweetheart. Believe that you can do it and you will be able to reach as far as your imagination takes you. Because experiences have no limits. Experiences hover about in an infinite place in which everything fits.

Don't suffer. Think now about yourself and about your own path.

Today, from this branch of the ash tree I admired so much when I was a little girl, I see myself in plenitude. I feel free, and I contemplate that which I was, with the serenity of one who has seen her life come full circle.

Life on Earth is a school, an apprenticeship. It is that place where we harvest experiences which guarantee our evolution. Not everything is easy, sweetheart. Consider that, and also believe that you have a right to be happy – that is why I tell you to search for happiness in everything, no matter the adversity you may face. It is important for you to know how to interpret the messages that life sends you, and you must cultivate positive values for you and yours.

You know? When I was on the Earth, suffering from the disease, the Alzheimer's that appeared to be grinding down my memories and my entire life, I had a very clear inner life. My mind became entangled, but inside, I felt myself bubbling with knowledge. I knew who you were, though my neurons could not manage to decipher the words to make you understand.

I knew my hands were becoming clumsy and useless, and that my words and my feet and even my physical being were deteriorating so quickly, anxious, perhaps, to leave that world which no longer belonged to me.

Because I was living in the other world, the world of Energies, and I was deciphering each color of the feelings. You remember, don't you? I always thought, ever since I was a child, that colors had their own scent. My pituitary always suggested that as the case. And now, here, where everything becomes feelings tied to the Essence, the smells are so sublime, so intense, as if everything were subtly connected, giving shape to the rose bed of dreams.

Sweetheart... do not ever suffer, even if you experience suffering. Think that, in the dance of life, you change partners. Sometimes you dance with pain, and pain makes you strong. You dance with sadness, and sadness makes a big enough space there for you so that, on the day when you dance with love, you can fill that place which once upon a time had been black and smelled of defeat. Then and only then, will you understand that pain and disappointment are necessary to make room for love, the feeling of love, which will always reach you.

Sometimes dreams are broken, but there will always be another dream. After all, is there anyone who can place limits on the imagination? My beloved daughter, the imagination is powerful. It keeps you away from what you do not desire, while it helps you to plot out your life. Because, when the goal goes in the direction that was plotted, that goal you dreamed of will come to you. The mind is powerful when it plans its course, and the rest of the road is defined by the strength of your feelings.

You know, when they diagnosed me with Alzheimer's, and after all that uncertainty, I left on that trip that I never took. My fantasy took me to the island. You told me I was doing the right thing when I began to fantasize about my trip, and you made it possible for me to dream everything I wished. And in my dream, there was that story of love I told you about only much later. And there I felt what it was to love again, though I never left the chair in my living room. And, believe me, I felt what I felt because the fairies helped me experience that brief but intense love story I never had.

I enjoyed Jorge's company, even though Jorge never existed for me, and I fantasized about him because I desired to live the here and the now, and reality did not allow me to do it, since by then ... the deterioration had already begun, mixing my story with the real story of my neurons.

126

The diagnosis had left me feeling defeated and not wanting to travel. I didn't even seriously consider it, even though in my story you gave me your blessing, and, shortly before I died, when I told you through my eyes that I had been loved in Tenerife and that I myself had loved, it was because my imagination made it possible for it to appear to be reality.

Don't let all your experiences go to waste, and let others know that not all is lost when life becomes trapped under the ground or upon the currents of the river. Because life continues just as a person who is ill continues, living behind his or her appearances.

Don't forget, dear Ana, my beloved daughter, that I was always there, though it seemed I had left.

Oh! And don't ever stop dreaming.